Conscious Awakening

Conscious Awakening

The Liberation of a Moonie and the Liberation of Humanity

Philip Sobul

AuthorHouse™
1663 Liberty Drive, Suite 200
Bloomington, IN 47403
www.authorhouse.com
Phone: 1-800-839-8640

© 2007 Philip Sobul. All rights reserved.
Celestial Mudra Publishing

No part of this book may be reproduced, stored in a retrieval system, or transmitted by any means without the written permission of the author.

First published by AuthorHouse 10/29/2007

ISBN: 978-1-4343-3319-3 (sc)

For more information about this title, please contact:
philip@sobulnow.com

Printed in the United States of America
Bloomington, Indiana

This book is printed on acid-free paper.

I dedicate this book to my wife Hyo Jung, My master Khan Bada, and spiritual teacher Eckhart Tolle without their support, magic, energy and inspiration I couldn't have written this book!

Table of Contents

Acknowledgements ix

Part I Peace on Earth

Chapter 1:   The Unification Movement
                and My Experience 3
Chapter 2:   The Divine Principle 21
Chapter 3:   Who Is Reverend Moon Anyway? 25
Chapter 4:   What Is a Messiah, and
                Do We Really Need One? 29
Chapter 5:   How the Collective Ego Infiltrates,
                Controls, and Dominates Organizations
                (Religious, Political, Corporate, or Other) 33
Chapter 6:   Jesus and Christianity 39
Chapter 7:   Islam 43
Chapter 8:   Living from Being and
                the Meaning of Nothing 49
Chapter 9:   Peace on Earth, Finally..55
Conclusion 63

Part II Conscious Awakening Now and Forever

Introduction		69
Chapter 1:	Trapped in the Mind, Time Dimension	75
Chapter 2:	Liberation in the Now, Immersion in Presence	79
Chapter 3:	Tipping the Scales	83
Chapter 4:	Freedom from Thought Possession	91
Chapter 5:	Freedom from Time	95
Chapter 6:	Freedom to Choose	99
Chapter 7:	Freedom to Do or Not to Do	101
Chapter 8:	Rewiring the Brain, Locking in the Gains	107
Chapter 9:	The Real Self	115
Conclusion		121

Part III Incarnations of Life: Search for our True Identity

Introduction		125
Chapter 1:	Altered States	127
Conclusion		149

Acknowledgements

I'd like to acknowledge and thank my spiritual teachers and guides. First of all, life itself is ultimately our own and everyone's spiritual teacher. But especially I'd like to thank Eckhart Tolle and the teachings of the power of now. I'd also like to thank Khan Ba Da and the work he's done with my wife, and ultimately her liberation as well. We are extremely grateful to these great contemporary spiritual teachers for what they have helped us with, as well as what is happening throughout humanity through these contemporary teachers as well as many others. The awakening of consciousness out of the dream of ego and into the present awareness of who we truly are.

Part I

Peace on Earth

Chapter 1

The Unification Movement and My Experience

Rarely has there been an organization movement—religious, spiritual, political—that has fostered so much opinion and emotion than the Unification Movement has over the past thirty years. I'm writing this book as a testimony and a witness to my experience during my time when I joined and I had my conversion experience; through the many years that I worked as a missionary, fund-raiser, and many other responsibilities directly, full time as a member; and subsequently after stepping back and separating my financial life from the movement many years ago and being able to take a look at—independently and rationally—what was going on in the movement, in the Church, both the good and the bad.

So the beginning of my story starts in 1974 before I went off to college. I had had a scholarship offered to me at a small liberal arts college in New England that I was planning to take—that was the fall of 1974. I was a restless kid; I grew up in the Midwest in a small town. There wasn't a lot to do. I lived in a normal family; although my parents had issues, I don't imagine they were very much different than any other family. So in that sense, I don't think I was from an unusually bad family. As a matter of fact, my mother is a very wonderful person, who suffered from bouts of depression here and there as I was growing up; and my father was a very good man with no real vices, but was emotionally shut off and found it very difficult to express love or emotion to his children; busy at work, busy making a living and doing his job.

As a kid, I developed a sense of longing for something real, something true. As a matter of fact, as I was dating in my youth, I would always chase girls away simply because I was too serious about the relationship at a young age. So there was something inside of me that was longing for—I don't know what you would call it; true love or a meaning or a purpose in life—something more than I felt in my family.

I also was a product of the late '60s and early '70s and did some experimentation with drugs; at the time marijuana, hashish, a little dabbling in LSD occasionally, but I never became addicted to any of them. But it did give me the experience of knowing that there are different states of consciousness than what we may be perceiving currently as we look at the world every day.

Having said that, and having spent the previous summer between my junior and senior year in high school traveling in Europe with a friend of mine for about six weeks, I planned on

Conscious Awakening

traveling the United States between my senior year in high school, when I graduated, and going off to college in September. So I set out on another adventure, another journey, looking for something; I didn't know what it was, but I knew that I needed to search. And I basically hitchhiked across the United States from the Midwest in five days, having various experiences with different people and different places, getting rides from here and there, and so on and so forth, which I don't want to really go into much in detail there, but it's not really important.

But I wound up on the coast of California in Santa Monica, one June afternoon, sitting on a beach, looking at the people on the beach, talking to some of them. One group of people came up to me and invited me to join them. They were going to travel up the coast, up to San Francisco. And I almost did that, except I felt there was one person in that group who was kind of the leader of the group that I just wasn't comfortable with. So I declined the invitation.

It was getting late in the day, and I went looking for some place to stay that evening. I walked up through the middle of town; Santa Monica at that point was an open air mall in the downtown, a walking mall. And I began to run into people from different organizations. I guess I ran into a couple of people who were affiliated with the Unification Movement; at that time they were called the One World Family. And my first impression when I met a couple of them who were male was, you know, Jesus, freak, get out of my face. I'm not interested.

Eventually, I sat down at a bench; and all of a sudden, I was approached by a young Finnish lady—rather attractive, not gorgeous, but you know, not too bad. And she walked up to me and looked straight at me; and for some reason, I was very open and nonresistant to her approaching me. Maybe because I was looking for a girl; I don't know what the reason was, but I was very open. We started talking about love and about life and so on and so forth. We probably talked nearly forty-five minutes. And then she said, "Would you like to come to our center this evening? We have dinner; we have a lecture."

I said, "Well, you know, I really don't have any place to stay." I had a backpack and some money in my pocket, and my plan was to go down to the docks and maybe sleep under the docks that evening. And she said, "Well, why don't you come to the center and have dinner with us. If you come, you have to listen to a lecture afterward, but at that point you can decide whether you want to stay or you want to go."

So I said, "Okay, I'm open-minded, what the heck." So we went. We got in a van with all the other people who were out on the streets witnessing at that point and we went to the center which was a very nice place. It was open air; there was a courtyard and some different houses that people stayed in, and then there was a room in the back where they taught.

It was a very nice atmosphere; people were very friendly and smiling, and it was kind of welcome after being kind of on my own for five days. I felt almost like at home in this atmosphere.

So we had dinner. The dinner was all right; I mean, it wasn't anything special, but it was food. I was hungry; I didn't have a lot of money. I had enough money that, I felt I could live for about six weeks if I was careful. But I was very judicious with my spending.

And then afterward, I heard the first lecture, which was an overview of the Divine Principle. It talked about the purpose of creation, the fall of man, the restoration of man, the mission of Jesus, the parallels of human history and the end days, and that this was a time when great changes were happening and that basically the coming of Jesus, it talked about that the second coming, was upon us. They didn't say who it was, they didn't say what it was, they just said it was upon us.

But more importantly, what I experienced during that lecture was an amazing sense of spiritual energy and openness that I was not really prepared for; but it was very, very profound. There were questions answered during that session that I had in the back of my mind about life, about Christ, the mission of Jesus; it was almost as if light bulbs were going off in my brain here and there. Little epiphanies that were just illuminating my consciousness. And I felt almost like transformed. Even in that first lecture. Definitely something was stirring in my consciousness that I had no idea and did not expect; but it was very, very profound.

This wasn't done in a coercive way; it was a simple lecture, full of nice people who were very clean cut and very wonderful. There was no brainwashing or psychological techniques that they talked about in the media over the years—nothing like that whatsoever.

So I told my spiritual mother, the Finnish lady that I had met, that I would like to…yeah, I'd like to stay and study further. This was very interesting, and so they invited me to a weekend workshop up in the San Bernardino Mountains outside of Los Angeles. And I went there on the weekend. At the retreat they went into a much more in-depth study of the Divine Principle, as well as praying and exercise and singing—a workshop with a number of people, a large number of people, which I think intensified the experience.

At that particular workshop, I felt even a greater sense of spiritual awakening, rebirth, what I would call in recently studying Hinduism in the last several years, something called a Samadhi experience—a sudden awakening, a growing sense of interconnectedness with all people, with life itself, with the universe, and my mind and heart became more and more peaceful and blissful and joyful. And I really felt that I had found something that was amazing. Certainly wasn't looking for this; my idea of what I was searching for was a relationship with a woman that could last and be true. All of a sudden, I'd found a spiritual awakening that I really hadn't been looking for. But it was there; it was obvious. It was profound. My whole sense of my innermost self had changed. And I felt such joy and peace that it's indescribable, the feeling that I had in that workshop in the San Bernardino Mountains.

So I went back to the center; having been immersed in this bliss—and it continued—it continued every day—and I began to participate in the activities of street witnessing and fund-raising, the activities that the members did in their daily life. So I decided to join the group.

I remember calling my parents and telling them this, and obviously they were distraught and wondered if I had gone off the deep end. Or, *What happened to you? What is the matter with you?* Their reaction was obviously very skeptical and very closed.

But I had this experience; and it had the effect—I would say in Christian terms, I felt that I was reborn. This was the rebirth experience that I had heard about growing up as a Christian. And it happened to me. And it was amazing.

So then a week or so later I went to another workshop that was seven days, and I began to feel at that workshop even a more profound sense of oneness with life and the universe and with all people and with God. It just kept growing and growing. That experience lasted for the next two months. Over a period of two months, we traveled throughout the West—Las Vegas, back to San Francisco, on a small witnessing team. We joined the group back in Las Vegas. This was a large group of missionaries, probably forty or fifty Europeans who were led by a German leader who I also felt a very close and deep relationship with as I got to know him. I really felt God's love and truth speaking through him profoundly.

Then it was discussed that Reverend Moon was going to be speaking in New York, Madison Square Garden, on September 18 and we needed to go to New York to help with the efforts, and we were going to drive across the country and we were going to fund-raise on the way, but we would get there in four or five days and we would be assigned different responsibilities to help make this great speaking event happen at Madison Square Garden.

So we arrived there about a month before the event, and I was assigned to the task of a fund-raising team, a group of about seven or eight of us, that we went off and left New York and went to Tennessee to raise money by selling candy and flowers and candles and things like that door to door and in shopping centers, at night outside of restaurants, even into bars. I could almost write a book about that experience in and of itself, the seven years I spent on the fund-raising teams after I joined the movement.

But this lasted for about a month, and it was good. I still felt that sense of peace and joy, but it had kind of lost its intensity to a certain degree because I was out in the public and working very hard and working for the mission. Helping to save the world, helping to bring the new truth to humanity.

So about a month later, we wound up back at Madison Square Garden. It was a very successful event. The place was packed; and it was a wonderful experience. Everything was great. But I had a longing to be back with the European missionaries whom I'd met and who had given me this wonderful experience—that I thought was the source of this experience. So we all went up to a property in Tarrytown, New York, which was the international headquarters at the time, to celebrate. There were people from all over the country there. I think there were ten missionary teams like this that I had hooked up with, that were traveling the different parts of the country. We celebrated and we recapped this successful event.

At this point I fully expected to rejoin that team and continue on with them; but all of a sudden, after the end of the celebration, there was a change of course. All of the American members who had joined these different missionary groups were now put into a new organization that was created and called the mobile fund-raising teams or MFT. And this was headed by a Japanese leader who was very close to Reverend Moon; it became his signature organization within the church. It was almost like the, you know, the Green Berets of the

Unification Movement. To go out on the fund-raising teams and work the way we worked for many, many years.

But anyway, getting back to the situation with me not reconnecting with the One World Family, which I had joined. Now I was involved with a new organization that wasn't really called a family. Now we were the Church and now we were organized into teams of fund-raising teams and we were under a completely different leadership, which was Japanese.

I remember feeling just empty and kind of like, this whole feeling of elation and joy was lost. But the memory of it was still there, very strongly. I had dedicated myself to this movement. And I said, "Well, you know, this is my opportunity now to grow and to sacrifice and to prove my worthiness to God by doing this." I spent the next three months fund-raising in various parts—back to Tennessee, then to Oklahoma, and all the way up till the end of the year.

I then remember a very difficult experience hit me on January 1, which in the Unification Church is called God's Day. Instead of New Year's Day, it's called God's Day, the first day of the year. I became very, very ill. This was in Tulsa, Oklahoma. My team leader at the time was getting more and more concerned about what was going on. There was a problem in my stomach, and I kept having this excruciating pain in my stomach. Finally the team leader said, "Well, we need to get you to a hospital."

They took me to a hospital in Oklahoma, and I basically had to have an emergency appendectomy performed on me because my appendix had started to rupture. It was actually infected with gangrene in my appendix.

I went through a very, very traumatic operation and very, very difficult recovery period in Oklahoma. I called my father since I was in the hospital, and the fund-raising team had to move on to new territory. I called my father and asked him if his insurance could cover me and if he could come to Oklahoma to meet me. And he did. He flew out to Oklahoma and we were there in Oklahoma and I was very, very sick. And it looked like it was going to be a month or so of recovery time. I asked the doctors in Oklahoma if I could go back to Ohio and stay with my parents in Ohio during the recovery time. And they said fine.

So we flew back to Ohio, my father and I, and my mother who had, you know, obviously been very worried about me for the almost six months that I had been away. I was very sick, but I started to recover; then all of a sudden, I had a relapse. There was an abscess in my intestines. I could not eat; nothing would go through. And I became very, very problematic. I had to go back into the local hospital in my hometown for another emergency operation, which again put me in the hospital for another ten days.

During that time, I couldn't eat, I couldn't drink, I had tubes in my wound, I had tubes down my throat. They had to completely dry me out and fill me full with high-powered antibiotics in order to kill any remnants of the gangrene that was in my system. So I was in the hospital for another ten days.

I got out again for a couple days, and then it started happening over again; but this time they just brought me back in, put me back on the tubes, and gave me more antibiotics. And about one month later, the end of January, I finally was able to leave the hospital and go back home.

I literally lost about ninety pounds during that process. When I walked out of the hospital, I had to basically learn to walk all over again. I looked like a survivor of Auschwitz— Nazi concentration camps. Totally, completely with no muscle mass—no, just basically skin and bones. Six-foot-two, 125 pounds, just really completely gone.

So I went back to my house, and I started my recovery and started to get my strength back and so forth and so on. I'm sure my parents, especially my mother, thought, *Well, you know, he's not going to go back to that crazy Unification Church or anything. Look what happened, he's certainly ill, you know. He will see the light and not go back.* Actually we had some arguments even while I was in the hospital, very emotional arguments about it because I told them I had every intention of going back.

Finally the time came when I was healthy enough to travel again, and I told my father, "Okay, I'd like you to put me on an airplane back to New York, I'm going to go back to the MFT headquarters and start to work again." And obviously my mother was extremely distraught; my father was—to give him credit—very fair-minded about it. I don't think he was happy about it, but he was not going to try to stop me from doing that. He respected my commitment and my opinion and said, "Okay, I'll bring you to the airport."

So I left that day, and I went out the door. My mother was holding my arm and crying and wailing and saying "Don't go; don't go!" And tears were running out of her eyes. And it was extremely difficult for me to leave, but I knew what I experienced and the profound nature of it; and I knew that I wanted to go back and continue my work with the movement.

So I went back to New York, and I started living—because I still needed some more recovery time—on that same property where the leader of the MFT lived, the small house on the property. It was a nineteen-acre property. And there I spent another month recovering until I was ready to go back into the fund-raising team.

But I remember going back and instead of being really welcomed with open arms and like, "Gee, you went through so much, you know, we're happy you're back," some people are like that. But the leaders were not. The leadership, especially the leader of the MFT, was very cold to me. And was almost like, "Well, why are you ill? Why are you sick? Why aren't you out doing your mission? Why aren't you dedicated to the point where even if you're ill, you're willing to go out and do your mission for God?" And this was the kind of attitude I had, and it was hard. It was a painful experience to go through that. But I figured, *Well, God's testing me to see what I'm really made of.*

And so I just let it go, I let it slide. I struggled with it for a while; I let it go.

And then finally I got back on the MFT and started fund-raising again and spent the next four or five years as a fund-raiser and also a team leader traveling throughout the United States, the South, the West, working very hard; seven days a week we would work. Six days we would work somewhere between fourteen and sixteen hours a day, and on Sundays we would work a six or seven-hour schedule and have some time to go to a restaurant or the movies for a little entertainment, a little break in the action.

Every day would start with prayer, a prayer service, and reading the Divine Principle or one of Reverend Moon's speeches, to inspire us to work hard and to do well and deepen our faith and our commitment. And quite frankly, I had many profound experiences when I was on these fund-raising teams, challenging my physical limitations, practicing faith, practicing the power of intention, never giving up, training myself to really believe and manifest that faith through my mission.

I also had tremendous experiences with the people I met, and learned about personalities and relationships and about myself, a tremendous amount of information about myself—what I could do, what I couldn't do, what my weaknesses were, what my strengths were. And as a leader, I developed an ability to speak and to guide the other members according to the faith. And I was—in the region I was in—mostly respected as a good leader. And it was a very, very interesting experience, those six or seven years; I forget how long it was.

And then one day, I was in Chicago. I had just been transferred from Florida to Chicago. I was with a new leader, a new regional director, who I thought was a maniac. I mean, he really was on fire. And at that point as a leader, I was only sleeping maybe two to three hours a night; and during the day, I would have to take breaks and sleep because the schedule was so severe we would work till 1 or 2 in the morning, go back to the center, sleep until 4, get up, go out, and fund-raise again before breakfast, then have breakfast, and then continue all day. And after seven years of this, of various degrees, I felt like I was losing my mind almost. Very, very difficult. I was struggling tremendously.

One day there was a phone call from New York and said that Reverend Moon was looking for some bodyguards for his property in New York. And I had been selected as a candidate to go and be interviewed for the position of bodyguard. So I went to New York and met with the leader of the MFT, the Japanese leader. He brought in a group of us to Reverend Moon's house, and we were interviewed and looked at and asked a few questions.

He chose four of us, and I became one of a team of bodyguards. We lived on the two properties where he at that point was staying most of the time between travels and public speaking engagements and things and managing the affairs of the movement throughout the world. Then I spent a good portion of five years there as a bodyguard, which wasn't just a bodyguard—that was my job at the property. I was also trained in martial arts, a style of tae kwon do and judo combination, and I was also trained as a lecturer for the Divine Principle and Unification Thought, the theories of the movement.

So our daily activities included eight hours to do personal care, which included sleep and hygiene, eight hours of being on duty as security guards on both properties, and eight hours of training, which would be lecture training, prayer, and also martial arts.

We also were living in the movement as brothers and sisters. There was no premarital sex while we were living as monks—as like nuns and priests. In other words, we abstained from any kind of sexual orientation, purifying ourselves, preparing ourselves for the future, to eventually be blessed in marriage through the church with a spouse, to create an ideal God-centered, purified family. And all the mission and the training was not just about saving the world but was also purifying ourselves to ultimately receive that blessing and have a family based on the teachings of the church.

And to me, it made a lot of sense. If you go back into the Divine Principle, the fall of man is symbolized by the story of Adam and Eve in the Garden of Eden eating from the fruit of the tree of knowledge of good and evil. This was in the Divine Principle terminology, symbolic of a premarital, self-centered, sexual relationship between Lucifer, the archangel who had become Satan, and Eve, who then tempted Adam to fall as well.

And this relationship happened prior to them achieving maturity and oneness with God. They were in the growth stage of their development when they had the external capabilities of having sexual intercourse but were not mature enough to really handle that. And they were tempted and subsequently fell and were cut off from the tree of life because of that issue. This is the teaching of the Divine Principle—man's perversion of love is the root of all evil. From godly, pure, totally selfless love, to self-centered, egotistical love is the core of human condition, the reason we are separated from God.

And so it just made total sense that through this practice, and through the purification, ultimately being able to be the blessing of God, we were restoring God's world and lineage, bringing new life into the world through this teaching, and that this was a central part of the changing of the world into God's world from the satanic world of hell.

And this was my experience as a bodyguard and my mission as a security guard at the property. And during that time, I saw firsthand Reverent Moon's lifestyle.

I saw his lifestyle, his experience. Even though he lived on a very nice property with tennis courts and swimming pool, I never once saw him play tennis or swim. As a matter of fact, I used the swimming pool and the tennis courts more than he ever did.

I also saw his schedule. He would keep a schedule of meetings with leaders from early morning till late at night—usually till 1 or 2 in the morning. During the time when he was under investigation for tax evasion and there were court cases and things going on, he had made a condition to go every morning up to the Holy Ground on the property and pray for an hour or so. And sometimes his wife would accompany him; sometimes it was just himself. At that time, I was on the night shift, and my job was to patrol around the property and make sure there were no problems. And I had my guard dog with me and many times I accompanied him from the front of the house all the way up to the prayer ground and I saw, in my opinion, a man of faith, a man of deep religious commitment, a man whose ideas and spirit and philosophy or spiritual teaching have the power to change the world. I was very impressed with him. And still am—to this day.

Eventually though I became tired of the mission. When I was at the front guard booth, I studied about many different things—business, financial markets, and other things. And there was some ambition developing me to go out and do something besides just being a security guard, although I knew it was very important from the church perspective. I really wanted to do more.

And eventually I made my way out of that mission and became involved in many of the business organizations within the church—with import/export businesses and so forth and so on.

And I also saw a lot of things when I was a security guard that were questionable and unsettling, especially when I saw his children get into trouble that caused me to wonder, you know, if this is really a true, the True Family as they purport to be; why are they experiencing similar difficulties with drugs and sex and various things? I thought this was supposed to be God's ideal family as a representation, an example of the way we were supposed to live. And it became increasingly problemsome for me to understand it.

Conscious Awakening

One explanation was well, you have a limited viewpoint, you still have your own fallen viewpoint; therefore, don't try to understand it because you won't. Don't judge. And I tried not to judge anyone; I figured that I went through struggles when I was growing up and they had to go through the same thing.

There were other problematic things though. I began to see the leadership that was under Reverend Moon and the very egocentric power games that they would play in the church—almost from the very leaders right under him, all the way down. And I began to see more and more of this throughout the movement. It was almost like when no one had any money, no one had any, you know, real power. Their ego took over, and everyone was struggling for position and recognition and favor and blessings from him and his family. And it became almost like the old TV shows I would see with my wife.

My wife happens to be Korean, and Reverend Moon engaged us during the Madison Square Garden marriage of two-thousand couples. And I would watch videos with her from Korea about the old kings and all the machinations of their court and their political situations and their deceptions and things like that. And I said, "Gee, it's very similar how this Church is organized in such a way; and there's all these things going on that somehow has no relationship with the organization I joined in California, the One World Family, where I had this peace and love and profound Samadhi or religious experience." Where did that all go? It was increasingly difficult for me to justify and rationalize it away.

Finally I wound up in a business organization with my brother-in-law who was the leader of the organization, and he eventually brought me up through the ranks. First of all, I never wanted to join it because I didn't want to be accused of nepotism; but he insisted strongly, almost to the point of fighting me about it physically, that I become a member of this business as a mission for the Church. And, ultimately, I worked my way up through the organization, the business organization, and became the general manager for about nine months or so. I was running the business and learning the business at the same time. I'd always been good at sales and marketing, but now I was learning administration and leadership management and so forth and so on. So it was a good experience. Not making much money, but there were a few perks; I had a company car and the prestige of being the leader of the business.

Then all of a sudden, after ten years, he fell out of favor and he was replaced by another leader who had been trying to take over this business from him for years. Finally he was successful. All of a sudden, I found myself in a position where I was the brother-in-law of the ex-leader who had been reassigned to another area of the country and back into the church side of the movement as a spiritual leader. And basically I was now the brother-in-law of the guy that was his enemy.

So I tried to hang on, and my brother-in-law encouraged me to stay there because he was going to try to get this position back. So he wanted me to stay there to make sure that he could come back within a short period of time. But increasingly it became extremely difficult to work with this person because in his mind, I was a marked man. I was still part of the old regime, and he wanted me out of there. So eventually I just resigned. And I said I'm sorry. And with the little money I was making, all of a sudden I was without a mission, without a job, without an income, and I had a wife to support.

I looked around in the Church for other businesses to work with. I went to Washington, D.C., I went to Connecticut. I looked around for real estate projects and other businesses. But nothing seemed to really fit. I knew a brother in the Church who was involved with our UN public relations organization; he was also working outside in a business in the insurance and financial planning business. So I went to him and said, "Gee, would it be nice? Could I get involved in this?" I had an interest in it.

So I went off and started my career in the financial services industry. But it was a profound change for me because now I had separated my financial life from my religious and spiritual life. And it gave me a sense of independence and objectivity that was obviously missing to a certain degree when I was working full-time in the mission—and looking to rationalize and justify the problems that I saw somehow and so forth and so on.

And that basically was my experience. During the years I've been involved with this career. I have distanced myself purposely, but I have become less and less involved in the movement, the central part of the movement, and more I would say an associate member for some time, not a core member. And now, I don't even consider myself to be a real member. I rarely participate in anything. I'll occasionally go to a Sunday service. I'll occasionally support something that I think is good that they're doing—such as the Middle East Peace Initiate. There are some things that they're doing in that area of the world that I think are very positive and very profound. And I've supported that with money and different things at times.

But by and large, I have a relationship of peaceful coexistence with the movement. I don't think the movement is bad; I don't think it's evil. I don't think that it has anything necessarily fundamentally wrong with the organization itself. It's just like any other organization; when you've got people and you've got money and you've got egos involved, there are problems.

This exists in every institution that you can look at throughout the world. The religious institutions, the political institutions, the corporate institutions, the community institutions, they all have the same problems. It isn't particularly an inherent problem of the Unification Movement or Reverend Moon per se; although the buck stops with him and he, being the leader, in my opinion, is responsible for what goes on, to a large degree. But it doesn't make this organization anything different than any other organization that's out there.

There are certainly people who have been in that movement or that Church for many, many years that are of the noblest character and the most sacrificial people that you can imagine. And they truly believe that they are on the leading edge of God's providence to change the world and restore God's kingdom today, in this world. And I respect that tremendously. They are people of exceptional character.

But I still think they're involved in a collective ego. Maybe their personal egos have been diminished because of all the sacrifice and all the selfless service that they have provided, but they're still part of a collective ego. Even though its teachings are, you know, one family of man, unify religions, unify philosophies, and create one world centered upon God—and those ideas are very noble—the practical reality is that the Church is very defensive when it's attacked. Every time anyone says anything bad or criticizes, there is a reaction of defense mechanism and ego from the leadership and from the members. Many of the members are the same way; it's a persecution complex basically.

And that can be very destructive because when members get involved in that kind of mind-set, they lose objectivity and they are not able to see clearly and be aware of the truth of what's happening.

So basically that sums up my experience in the Unification Movement. I could go into each one of these segments in much greater detail, but that's not the purpose of this book. This is my perspective. I think it's a very fair and balanced perspective; I have seen this movement and this Church from the top all the way to the bottom and from the inside and the outside. And I've experienced the greatness and the profound nature of it in the marrow of my bones. And I've seen some of the significant problems and issues associated with it. And that's really what I would like to witness to.

Chapter 2

The Divine Principle

Basically we're talking about the unification teaching or the Divine Principle. In 1936, Reverend Moon received a revelation from Jesus, a vision about the new age that was dawning. Jesus in a vision told Reverend Moon that he wanted him to lead the restoration, or reformation, of God's kingdom at this time on earth. Over a period of time, he received a revelation called the Divine Principle, which is in many ways a clarification of some of the mysteries of the Bible as well as other spiritual teachings. It has elements of Taoism, Buddhism, and a lot of Christian scripture and Christianity and biblical support. So the Divine Principle was the basic teaching. Also, Reverend Moon's speeches from many, many years are filled with many maps and signposts to the truth.

Many members experienced awakening and transformation for some time, only to get lost ultimately in the collective ego system—proclaiming to be the center of God's providence, which is what a lot of other Christian denominations claim: that they are the way, that you must join their organization, otherwise you're not part of this new age.

They turned themselves into another religious organization stuck on their own signpost, worshipping their leader as god. Most members I know and keep contact with do not feel happy or liberated; they feel like they're in prison. And in one sense, they are in prison in their own form of their own collective ego or consciousness. But so is most of humanity, in one form or another. This isn't a peculiarity of the Unification Church; they need to realize that no one is building God's kingdom. It is within all of us already as Jesus taught. No one really has a monopoly on that either.

Humanity needs liberation. It is very important to understand that the teachings, any spiritual teaching, is not the truth itself. No words or language can contain the truth; they are just road maps or signposts pointing to the ultimate reality. The egotistic consciousness wants to imprison the truth so it can control life and survive. Most religion or spiritual teachings and their followers make the mistake of turning signposts into belief systems and ultimately their own egotistic prison. The Bible is not the truth but a beautiful road map filled with many pointers or signposts. It is not reality itself.

Ultimate reality, the one life or God or whatever name or label you want to put on it, could never be contained in an intellectual concept. Even science has the same problem, trapped in the level of egotistic thought and narrow, limited perspective. Science is its own religion, masquerading in the guise of academic credibility.

Humanity needs liberation. Liberation from the egotistic mind and its psychological addiction to past and future. That liberation exists within the now. The one eternal, timeless moment we all experience as our lives—the present awareness—is here and now and never leaves us and has been with us forever. The one place where the ego will suffocate. . I have basically one message for Unificationists throughout the world, and that message is really simple and clear. There is no "them." Life is not about us and them. Life is not about inside members and outside people. There is only us, one humanity. One life, one consciousness, and one liberation. And as Jesus said in the Gospel of Thomas, "Look within yourselves, and you will find that, if you know where to look."

Chapter 3

Who Is Reverend Moon Anyway?

Religious leader, prophet, messiah, charlatan, brainwasher, head of an international conglomerate of wealthy, powerful organizations, true parent, true father of humanity. You name it, people have opinions regarding who Reverend Moon is.

Ultimately, Reverend Moon is nothing more than pure consciousness. Ultimately, pure awareness. Just like you and me. Just like all of us, at the deepest level of our being, we are all being, consciousness, and bliss, or the Hindu term *sachitnanda*. We are all one. One fabric of the cosmos, of the universe.

Scientists today have proven the fact that there is no separate entity in the world, that everything is interconnected. All energy, all life, all humanity. And the separateness that we believe and feel is just an illusion. The great traditions of Buddhism, Hinduism, and others have taught this concept and this idea and lived this for years. For centuries.

So ultimately, who is Reverend Moon? Depends on the perception of your own consciousness. For most great spiritual teachers, their greatness comes in their ability to reflect back to the perceiving person themselves. This is true of Jesus. This is true of Buddha. The genius of any spiritual teacher, enlightened human being, pure conscious awareness, is in the ability of that that teaching or that person to reflect back to who they are.

Ultimately there is a much more important question to ask than who Reverend Moon is or who Jesus is or who Buddha is or who Ramana Maharshi is or any great sage or enlightened person that we may or many not know of. The most fundamental question is, Who am I? Who are we? And who am I? Do we know ourselves at the level of being, at the level of I am? The I-am-ness of life. Before I think, before I do anything, I am. Before I am this or that—a doctor, a lawyer, a father, a criminal, a patient, a sick person, a beggar, an advisor—I simply *am*. Which is the first person pronoun of the verb *to be*. To be is I am.

So what is humanity's problem anyway? What is it that makes so much madness in the world? That allows people to commit atrocities and indignities and murder? To pollute the planet and all kinds of problems that you see daily on the news and throughout human history and throughout the twentieth century? What is this dysfunction?

Ultimately, in the words of Eckhart Tolle, it is the problem of identification with the mind-made ego itself. We don't know ourselves as the awareness, the I-am-ness of life. We know ourselves only as the form, the thing, the mental concept, the story in our brains that keeps incessantly repeating itself on and on and on. That perceives the world as hostile—that perceives the world as us and them.

And as long as humanity remains in the grips of that egotistic consciousness, there will never be peace on earth, there will never be the paradise that this world was meant to be.

So it becomes a problem of the personal ego and also the problem of the collective ego as the personal ego controls and dominates organizations of all kinds. And unfortunately I can say that is a phenomenon that is still very prominent in the Unification Movement. But that's not their problem alone. It's true of any organization.

Look at communism. What happened to communism? They had the idea of no personal property. Sharing the world with each other. One humanity. Brothers and sisters in the struggle. Liberation from the horrors of capitalism. Paradise on earth. And where did it go? Decades and decades of misery and destruction and human degradation and murder. Why?

The idea wasn't the problem. There was no shift of consciousness away from identification with the mind and with the ego. So it was destined to fail. As any organization will be destined to fail as the collective ego gets stronger and stronger and becomes more and more mad and mad.

So who is Reverend Moon anyway? The founder of this movement, the founder of the Unification Church, the founder of numerous other political and business organizations. His ideals are noble: the kingdom of heaven on earth, God's world, the end of suffering, the end of war and establishment of peace, tranquility, beauty. But ultimately, unless that organization or any other organization can transcend the collective ego and become pure consciousness, it's also destined to fail.

Chapter 4

What Is a Messiah, and Do We Really Need One?

The concept of the messiah has been around for centuries, for millennia. The Jewish people, the Hebrews, were waiting for the messiah for hundreds of years. The liberator. The one who will take them to the promised land.

In Christian terminology, a *messiah* is the way, the truth, and the life. The way to God. The way to salvation. They way to have eternal life. The person to believe and follow. The one who will take up the cross. The opening to the eternal dimension.

But ultimately that dimension exists in all of us. Again, the concept of the messiah. Ultimately this dimension exists in all of us. And the true role of a spiritual teacher is to help us uncover that which keeps us from realizing who we truly are at the deepest level. So if you equate ego and consciousness or sin or fallen nature or ego identification with darkness, the messiah, the guru, the spiritual teacher is the person who shines the light of consciousness and awareness on that within us that obscures our divine nature. And helps us realize that we are not evil, that we are not sinful, that we are not guilty, that we are a product of thousands of years of conditioned egotistical thinking. That at the deepest level, we are pure conscious awareness. We are the light.

So ultimately, even the messiah cannot save us. Nothing from outside of ourselves can save us, ultimately, absolutely. We must save ourselves. And when that happens, there is no more need for a messiah. There is no need to elevate any one person to the role of God, to the idol, to something other than what we already are, each one of us. In that sense, enlightenment is nothing special. Enlightenment does not mean elevated place, better than others, revered, different, out of touch, out of reach. We can never be enlightened. We can never be divine. We can never be pure consciousness. We are condemned to this sin, to this sinful world, to the ego.

So if anyone says "Here is the messiah," don't go that direction. The Bible says in Revelation, "He is here or he is there, he is over there." In the last days there will be many false prophets and messiahs. How can you recognize if you have a pure spiritual teacher or not?

Look at the ego. Is everything centered around that person's ego? Or is that person, that spiritual teacher, egoless? Humble? Pure? Because a true spiritual teacher is either on the way or is completely liberated from egotistic consciousness and the conditioning of the human mind.

Once again, at that point, do we really need a messiah? The ultimate goal of the messiah, if there was one, would be to eliminate the messiah by helping everyone elevate themselves to who they truly are—pure consciousness, pure awareness, which also is peace, compassion, and love in its truest sense. Not the egotistic, grasping, self-centered love that dominates the media and our human relationships.

Chapter 5

How the Collective Ego Infiltrates, Controls, and Dominates Organizations (Religious, Political, Corporate, or Other)

Beside each one of us struggling and dealing with the ego is the mind-made illusory consciousness that keeps us from realizing our true identity. This then magnifies and intensifies as a collective ego when it comes to organizations. If you look at the history of organizations, whether they be religious, political, corporate, community, without exception they are dominated by a collective egotistic consciousness that is simply a manifestation of each personal ego working in a group.

And the reason for this is very simple. Unless the individuals within an organization, and especially the leadership in an organization, is able to disidentify themselves from that egotistic mind-made self and realize on the deepest level of their true nature of who they are as enlightened pure consciousness, all organizations are doomed with the same problem and the same set of circumstances. And it repeats itself over and over again.

Let's look at the situation in the Middle East for an example. An ancient struggle dating back to the time of Abraham between Ishmael and Isaac. Deeply rooted animosity and hatred fueled by the egotistic sense of self that has perpetuated itself throughout history in one form or another and is currently manifested as the Middle East conflict between the Israelis and the Palestinians. Both sides are victims, and both sides are absolutely convinced that they are right and the other is wrong. And it's the struggle for territory, autonomy, that is much more than just a struggle over land. It's basically a struggle on the level of ego of who is right and wrong.

One side attacks, the other side stiffens, and the sense of ego strengthens. That's the very nature of it because the ego knows it's not real ultimately, it's just an illusion. It's always looking to create enemies, someone to be against, someone to attack.

It's really quite simple. Because of the problem of the individual being identified with ego, with the mind. Not only identified but literally possessed by that entity. In an effort to strengthen its sense of self, to prove its own existence which is ultimately an illusion, we join organizations, we join religious institutions, we join political organizations. We're members of this, that, and the other thing. And that in and of itself is not bad; it's perfectly normal to live in community and harmony with others. But when we do that in order to strengthen our sense of self as a need of egotistic consciousness, we then ultimately create madness on a collective level.

And you can see that clearly in governments, in religious institutions, in the corporate world; it is dramatic. Everyone trying to prove that they're better than the other, to get ahead. Get up on the Joneses. Not just to keep up with the Joneses—but to get up on the Joneses. To get that promotion, to get ahead of my colleague, to beat the competition. To control the wealth, the form. To dominate the form. To be master of the universe.

And when you look in the eyes of these leaders, especially the business leaders and the political leaders, and you looked in the depth of their soul, what do you see? It's certainly not peace; it's certainly not the joy of being—it's the obsession with egotistic consciousness. Period. It's the obsession of trying to inversely strengthen its sense of identity which ultimately is futile because at the center of ego, there's no substance. It's a great black hole feeding on achievement, feeding on its own sense of self. Never satisfied ultimately. Going back and forth between pain and pleasure, achievement and failure—the duality of life. In Buddhist terms, its called *samsara*, the endless cycle of karma.

So you see it everywhere. You see it especially in religious institutions. We have the truth. We know a better way. If you don't believe like we do, you are not saved. You are condemned to hell. Follow us. Give us your mind, give us your work, give us your money. Give us all that you have so that we can be stronger as a collective ego.

The ultimate purpose of religion is to end religion, to take us from the level of thought and form and religious dogma into the realm of being and knowing. But the collective ego doesn't want that. They don't understand that. They have to keep gathering more people, gathering more money, gathering more power, building bigger edifices to ourselves, to our dominance of the truth.

And those who are not believing like us, let's oppose them. Or better yet, let's attack them. Let's destroy them. They're heathens, they are not God's chosen people—God will reward us if we kill them. What madness.

But that's not any more mad than "If you don't believe like me you're going to hell. We know what is right and wrong; we know what's good and evil. We're good, and you're evil. We're on God's side. So let's go kill the evil in the world. That'll make us feel more righteous. Then we'll dominate even more." It's also madness ultimately. This is not the road to peace. Look at the Middle East. Thousands of years of madness, struggling over one piece of land. Struggling between one egotistic collective against another.

If we know ourselves, truly who we are, the entire universe is ours. We don't need to fight over one piece of land; we need to share the world and the universe with each other. Why be limited? Why be separate? For what reason? It's also madness.

You are not separate from each other; you are one life, one family, one humanity. Don't fight anymore. Put down your weapons. Then put down your egos. Learn to be. Find the peace in that place where there is no conflict, where there is no us and them. Do not commit acts of violence against yourselves in the name of God, in the name of Allah, in the name of Jehovah, in the name of Brahmin. This is also madness.

The collective ego works in other ways. In the world of sports. Rivalry weekend. My team is going to beat your team. Surely we don't have to give up rivalries, do we? How do you feel when your team loses? Are you depressed? Are you angry? Do you resent the other team? This is collective ego. The Red Sox and the Yankees. Ohio State, Michigan. Texas, Oklahoma. Florida, Florida State. Collective ego.

We need to recognize within ourselves, within our organizations, within our political system, within our religious institutions, in every aspect of humanity, we need to shine the light on the darkness and let it go. Let's just let it go. Let's move on. Let's be humble. Let's be sincere. Let's be ourselves at the fundamental level—free, of the mind.

The mind is not its own master. It is a servant of being. It should be used creatively, productively, positively. But that has to emanate from deep inside who we truly are.

And on the collective level where there is leadership, it must come from that leadership. We need that kind of leadership. We don't need more egotistic madness.

No one is immune; no country is immune. No organization is immune. We are all guilty of it; let's be honest. We are all guilty on the individual level, on the collective level. But what is guilt? Guilt is just another way the ego tries to cover up our pure consciousness. It's another poison to who we are. So let's forgive each other; let's forgive ourselves. And let's move on. Let's let the power of these organizations, the collective power of pure consciousness working together, create a new world of great beauty, of great innovation, of justice, peace, and love. Not of greed and strife and suffering.

So the collective ego is an extension of the individual ego. It's a way for the individual ego to gain more power, to establish itself more firmly in the control of our lives. But that's not who you are. We need to uncover who we are. We need to find our identity beyond the mind. This is liberation. This is freedom. This is peace. This is joy. This is love at the essential level. It is a world beyond your wildest dreams. Let go of the old world, as individuals egos, as a collective ego. Let it go.

Chapter 6

Jesus and Christianity

Who is Jesus Christ, anyway? It's a question that's been asked through the ages, through the centuries of time since he was born, lived, taught, was crucified and died on the cross, buried and resurrected. Was he the messiah? Was he God himself? A son of God? The prophet? A heretic? A charlatan?

Ultimately, Jesus Christ is pure consciousness, with no egotistic covering. The light of the world, the light shining through, the light of pure consciousness. One with the divine. And nothing special. And example of who we were all meant to be. The second Adam. Brother of Buddha and Mohammed, as well as other enlightened humans in the past.

Let's not turn him into a golden calf. Moses went to the top of the mountain to get the Ten Commandments from God. And when he came down, the people were worshipping a golden calf. What did Moses do? He destroyed it.

When we turn Jesus into a golden calf, we put him in a prison. It's exactly where the ego wants him. It's over there, up there. To be worshipped as a god. Different than us. We are not like that. We can never be like that. Poppycock. We were meant to be, and we were created by the same power, by the same pure consciousness. We are all pure consciousness, divine consciousness. We are just asleep at the wheel. We need to wake up.

Jesus was fully awake. He knew who he was. He manifested all the characteristics of that pure consciousness. And ultimately he made the ultimate sacrifice for all of us. Not as I will but as thy will. It's a total surrender to the now, to the moment, to the eternal life. To the opening, to the divine. He didn't display any weakness in the garden. That's poppycock.

So where is Christianity today? And I'm talking about all forms of Christianity. The Catholic, the Protestant, the various denominations, fragmented, cut up into pieces. Bickering about who's right and who's wrong. The collective ego.

We don't need that anymore. We don't need any self-righteous preachers. We don't need any pedophile priests. We don't need any theological philosophies. We just need to know who we are in our essence. Just like Jesus did.

We really have no excuse, in one sense. But when you're unconscious, you're unconscious. Jesus said, "Forgive them for they know not what they do." So we need to forgive ourselves because we know not what we do. And that the time for forgiveness is over. Let's not create the conditions that we need to be forgiven for. The pure consciousness will forgive us when we wake up to who we are.

Christianity needs reform. It needs to realize that the purpose of religion is to end religion on the level of mind and form. The Tao Tai Ching says that if you can talk about it, that's not it. The truth is beyond the pointer; the truth is beyond the signpost. The truth is within us. I am in the Father, and the Father is in me. And in you, and I in you. The Father is in the rocks, the trees, the forest, the streams, the animals, and ultimately in each human being. It's in there. It's in there.

Let's stop the madness. Let's move on. Let's fulfill the mission of Christianity to unite the world. Not under Christianity. Under pure consciousness. Beyond thought and form. We all are welcome. The Moslem, the Hindu, the Buddhist, the Sufi, the Jew. Our family. Our heart. We don't need belief systems anymore. Heaven is here in your midst. It's not a reward for a belief system. It isn't seventy-two virgins waiting in paradise when I die. Jesus said the kingdom of heaven is at hand. It's here and now. It's in your midst. Wake up.

And what do we do, The collective ego? We put him to death. It wasn't the Jews who killed Jesus. It was all of us. This isn't a personal problem for any people.

The ego is everyone's problem, all of humanity. And that's what killed Jesus. The ego didn't want what Jesus could bring, it didn't want the kingdom of heaven on earth, it didn't want world peace, it didn't want the joy of being, it didn't want any of it. And then we got this result. The tragedy of the cross and the glory of the resurrection. The opening to the divine. The salvation of humanity.

But that opening is available to all of us as we face our daily challenges in life. Jesus said you have to take up your cross and follow. And in the egotistic conscious level, there are challenges that are constantly presented to us on the level of form. The question is, do we fight them? Or do we surrender to them? Do we allow those challenges? They're seemingly difficult situations. Those little deaths, the losses of our lives, when what we want and expect doesn't happen the way we wanted and expected it to. The dead piece of fish. The accident. The lost gift. The lost job. The death of a family member. The death of a child.

We can resist it because we do not like pain. We just like pleasure. Or we can accept what Buddha said, the suchness of life, and align ourselves with life.

When Jesus was asked to sacrifice himself, he didn't say no. He surrendered to the moment. Not as I will, but as thy will. When the will of life knocks on your door, are you going to lock the door? Or are you going to allow it to come in, whatever it is? Because whatever it is, is what you need, no matter how the mind judges it. In whatever form life takes. Let's trust that. Because beyond that door, there's peace. Beyond that door is pure consciousness. Beyond that door is who we are. Let's walk through the door no matter what the pain might be.

Chapter 7

Islam

This is the meaning of Islam. Islam means to surrender.

Now I don't know much about Islam, intellectually. I know I see in the world a great spiritual tradition of love and adoration for Allah, which is God, pure consciousness, the one life. In that sense, Jesus was Islamic. Surrendered to God. God's will be done. Then Mohammed came along and did the same thing and inspired millions to live a life of faith and devotion to God. It's beautiful.

However, there is one aspect of so-called Islam that is not

really Islam. It's just the ego's way of distorting and perverting the truth. The jihad (the jihadist) is not emanating from the joy of being. It's again the collective ego. But this time the collective ego is full of rage and unbelievable negative energy where there are no laws or rules to follow at all except one. To kill the heathen, purge the world. Once again it's egotistic madness, guised as a holy war—it happened before, centuries and centuries ago. The Crusades, the battle for Jerusalem, the battle for the Holy Land, which continues today. The same egotistic madness. The same problem. The same challenge.

There is no solution on the level of mind and ego and form unless there's a shift in consciousness, away from mind and form, and into pure consciousness, awareness, being, presence. But the doorways are everywhere in that state of consciousness.

Whenever you're faced with a challenge in life, let it be. It doesn't mean you can't change the situation; but at that moment, when that challenge faces you, when that problem crops up, embrace it. And digest it. Move through it. And open the door to that new dimension. Do not resist. To resist life is madness. To resist the suchness of life is insanity. It's the food that ego lives on. It's the source of the ego's power. The ego cannot exist within you; it will lose all of its power if you surrender to the now. The suchness of life. Embrace it, whatever it is. Allow it to be. Digest it. It may be a great meal, and it may be bitter medicine. But life itself only gives you what you need. If you believe otherwise, it's delusion.

You are not separate from life; there is no "my life." There is no "my spiritual life." There is no "my story." There is just one life. You are life itself. Become aligned with it, become its friend. Ultimately, it means becoming friends with yourself. Ultimately, it means losing the myself and realizing that I am. We are not two; there isn't "I" and "myself," there is just "I." The one life, pure consciousness. There is no "my life," "my spiritual life," "my political life," "my career." This is ultimately delusion. It's ego's way of separating us from life.

So Islam is profound. Islam, which means to surrender, is the secret to life. Connect to it. We are like the most magnificent TV. The latest flat screen plasma television. But we're not plugged in to the power. That is Islam. That is Jesus. That is Buddha. They were plugged in. And they manifest all the wonders of life.

And you have that in you already. You don't need to become any more than you are already. Life is not imperfect; life is perfect. Jesus said, "Be ye therefore perfect as your heavenly father is perfect." He didn't say try your best and when you ultimately stumble and fall and never live up to that expectation, I'll forgive you. Don't make excuses. It is not human weakness and human frailty. Humanity is divine. You are divine. Your mind is divine comedy, and life is divine opportunity. That is Islam. That is Christianity. That is Buddhism. That is Catholicism. That is Sufism, Janism. Bahai. Unificationism. Hare Krishna. Hinduism. That is science. That is quantum physics. It's all in there. Why do we need to label, categorize, identify, separate, cut up, butcher one life? It's madness.

It's time to stop. The party's over. It's time to pull the curtain on that drama. There's a new show opening just down the street. Let's all go to the new show. You'll be surprised at what you'll find. Do not fear anything. The only thing we need to fear is fear itself. Fear doesn't exist; it's an illusion.

There is no death. Then why are we so afraid of death? If we are identified with our ego, the little pygmy in us that knows it isn't real knows about its own black hole of unreality. Of course we're afraid of death. But look at the leaves of the trees. Look at the animals. Are they afraid to die? Do they have mental and psychological problems when they are confronted with their own imminent death? They surrender to the will of life. They surrender to the impermanence of form without any problem, without any misery, without any suffering. Are you ready to die?

When I was a child, I watched a movie called *Little Big Man* which starred Dustin Hoffman. He was a white boy born of Caucasian ancestors who somehow wound up living with the Indians in the great West, the days of Buffalo Bill. And the slogan, the motto, of those Indians when they woke up every morning was "Today is a good day to die."

When we wake up every morning, let's not look for something, not just look for pleasure and avoid the pain. Pain and pleasure are the different sides of the same coin. You cannot escape both sides in the world of mind and form. There's no escape. There is no escaping the death of the mind and form. It was born, and it will die. It's a temporary expression of eternal life. So let's not fear death. Let's wake up every morning and say, "Today is a good day to die." Today I surrender to life. Die to the moment, die to the past. Die to the problems. Let them go. Ultimately surrender our physical life when the time comes. When that moment is now, then do it in beauty and grace and peace and love and gratitude for all that life has given you while you were temporarily masquerading as your form. The masquerade party's over. Time to take off the mask.

When you can face death in this way, that's liberation. That's peace. That's what Jesus meant when he said I have overcome the world. People thought he was crazy. He had no power, he had no money, he had no political clout, he had no armies. How did he overcome the world? He transcended death. He totally disidentified from the forms of the world and ego and realized who he was and let that light shine forth.

Today there are many spiritual teachers who are also showing us the way. Not just one. Not just one messiah, one savior. Like I said before, we have to save ourselves. But the power is within us.

The Gospel of Thomas, verse 70. It's curious how that isn't in the Bible, the teachings of Jesus were a lot more than what's in the traditional Bible today. The collective ego suppressed it hundreds of years ago. Buried it. But it was found in 1945 in Egypt.

Ultimately, the ego will destroy itself. Let's help it along. The truth always comes out eventually.

Chapter 8

Living from Being and the Meaning of Nothing

Thinking and doing, doing and thinking. I think, therefore I am. I must do something in order to become something. This is the common sense normal consciousness in today's world. Wrapped up in doing. Striving to be something. Trapped in form. Prisoner of the little me, the little egoistc mind, that because of its insecurity of knowing that it's not real, is obsessed with doing, getting someplace, going somewhere. Arriving at some future moment where I have made it. Never,

never getting there. Always winding up empty and frustrated, and thinking that, "Well, if I just do more, if I just think more, if I just work harder, if I just gain more wealth, more status, more of something, that ultimately I will find myself."

Ultimately this is the fundamental dysfunction of humanity. Lost in thought. Lost in the world of form. Identification and attachment to the forms of the world, whether it be our body, our appearance, our thoughts, our emotions; obsessed with living in the world of form. And failing to recognize that we truly are as the being, or the I-am-ness out of which our thinking and our doing comes from.

So what is primary? Doing or being? Actually, being is primary. Any thinking and doing that is not rooted in being, that doesn't emanate from being, is ultimately wasted time and energy. And leaves us feeling empty and spent. So doing and thinking must first of all come from being. And how do we know, or how do we feel that being, that I-am-ness? We have to understand that we are not our thoughts, we are not our physical form, we are not our emotions. But we are the awareness, or the I-am-ness in which those thoughts, those emotions, in which our life unfolds.

Just like a room. If you take a look at the consistencies or the things that make up a room, there are really two dimensions. If you look at the room I'm sitting in now, there are the things in the room—the lamp, the bed, the walls, the wallpaper, the ceiling, the television, the light, the door. But there's something more. There's the space in which those things or those forms exist. Without the space, there would be no room. There would be no things in the room. Now this is true of ourselves. Without the consciousness, without the unmanifested awareness that we are, there would be no form. There would be no body, there would be no mind, there would be no thoughts.

This level of being or I-am-ness or pure consciousness is the fundamental ground of all existence, of all form. This is being. To be. I am. This is primary.

Conscious Awakening

How do we develop a sense of being? We have to strip away all the things that being is not. We have to peel it away. We have to disidentify ourselves from the forms. This is the fundamental exercise of meditation. To observe, to be aware. To rest in our own being. To watch our feelings, our thoughts, our emotions, our sense perceptions. One step removed from them, as the witness. As the awareness. And as that happens, as we peel away the layer of the outside world of form and the body, the mind, the thoughts, the emotions, we peel that all away and we realize I am not that. What remains is nothing.

Now you might say, "Well, I am something. I am not nothing. I don't want to be nothing." But that's what you are. At the fundamental level, you are no thing. And the ego doesn't like that. If you think about that concept—I am nothing—the ego will react to that. That doesn't feel very good; I don't like that.

So ultimately to find being, we need to become comfortable with being nothing. We need to become comfortable with being nothing. We need to be comfortable with having nothing. We need to be comfortable with nothing. And when you start to feel that comfort, when you lose that desire to have, to possess, to become, to do, to strive for, to achieve, and you start to be comfortable with nothing, you start to feel being at its fullest.

Because there's something there, actually. It isn't a void. It isn't a nihilistic extension. There's a peace there; there's a serenity. There's a sense of well-being. There's a sense of God there. The one life, life itself, the essence of life is resting in that nothing. Because indeed it is no thing. It is the unmanifested. Before there is anything, there is nothing. In Buddhism it's called "Form is emptiness and emptiness is form."

Now to the mind that sounds crazy. How can form be emptiness and emptiness be form? But in reality, without the emptiness, or without the nothing, without the unmanifested, there could be no manifested. Without the eternal, there could be no temporal or impermanent, transient form.

So this is what's important. Humanity as a whole learns to live from being. Learns to think and do, not for its own sake, for the sake of the little me, the little mind, the little egotistic consciousness; but we learn to transcend that egotistic consciousness, mind-made self, and live and emanate our living and doing and thinking from the state of being. Our deep-rooted sense of self.

All the great spiritual traditions of history point to the same thing. We are not, but we think we are. We are suffering from a fundamental identity crisis on a spiritual level. And because we don't know who we are, or we have a false sense of identity, we're mistaken, we think we can find ourselves in the things of the world. My car. My house. My children. My life. My pain. As if we were able to own life. Which ultimately is delusion. There is no "my life." There is life, and that's what we are—one life. Interconnected.

Twenty six hundred years ago, The Buddha taught about the interconnectedness of the world, about the cosmos, the universe. All things of the world are ultimately connected in one field of energy. There is no separate anything, there is no self. Buddha said there is no self that's separate from the whole. There is no mind-made self. There is no ego. It doesn't exist. Ultimately, it's a delusion.

Because we lost that sense of interconnectedness, become trapped in thinking and doing, an obsession with thinking and doing, we view the world as separate, as hostile. It's like a game of survival. Therefore, anything's okay as long as it supports my survival. Even if I need to hurt someone, even if I need to steal or cheat. Or even kill something. It's okay. If we truly understood that we are all one, that we are all connected, if we truly understood in the marrow of our bone, in the depth of every cell of our body, in the depth of our soul, who we are as one life, hurting someone or killing someone would be like killing ourselves. No one would do it. It would be impossible to harm. And instead of this sense of fear and survival instinct and viewing everything as a hostile world, to be fought out and to be feared, deep love and compassion, unity, peace would be the normal thing.

Living from being or conscious living is what humanity needs more than ever. Without it, things are only going to get worse. We live now in the age of super technology. Man's ability to do things and create things in a destructive manner has reached its height. With the push of a button, we could annihilate ourselves.

Living from being, it's what we need.

Chapter 9

Peace on Earth, Finally

Throughout human history, humanity has been longing for peace. The cry of the human soul throughout the history of humanity is for world peace. End of conflict. The end of distress. The end of war. Why has it not happened? Why is the madness continuing and seeming to get worse and worse with every passing year, with every passing decade, with every passing century? Why do human beings continue to inflict tremendous atrocity and misery on each other when in every heart and every mind throughout humanity there is this cry for peace?

Philip Sobul

There is only one answer. Peace is impossible as long as humanity is identified with the egotistic consciousness. Quite simply, the ego does not want peace because peace can only be found when we have stopped identifying ourselves as the little mind-made me. The tape recorder in our brain, the life story, and realize who we truly are—divine, pure consciousness that would allow us to see all humanity as one, interconnected in one energy and one mind, and in one heart.

It's only in that place we can find peace. Each human being needs to have peace themselves within the depth of their soul. Peace can only come from that place, the divine place in all of us. Peace can only come from being. It can ever come from doing or thinking. There is no treaty, no peace agreement, nothing that can be written on paper that will never bring lasting peace. No constitution, no treaty, no agreement between countries, between political systems, between religions that will ever bring lasting peace.

So you may wonder, When will this ever end? And can it ever end? The madness that we see daily on our television sets throughout the world. Not only as manifestations of war between nations and conflicts between peoples and disagreements or conflicts between religions. When will it ever end?

Fortunately, as the craziness gets worse and worse, there is something else happening. On a scale that's never been seen before until recently, the phenomenon of the flowering of consciousness has only happened in a few isolated individuals throughout human history. Buddha, Jesus Christ, Mohammed, and a few other saints and sages, from India and throughout other spiritual and religions traditions. And the effects of their lives had been felt greatly throughout human history. The rising of that pure enlightened consciousness shown in all of these people has kept humanity from annihilation.

But it has not been enough for humanity to transcend the ego, the identification with form. The identification with thought. We have not realized life as being life here and now. In this moment. Eternally living in the moment. The timeless dimension where past and future psychologically have no power whatsoever. It's the fundamental nature of the ego to hate peace because peace on that level means the annihilation of the ego. Ultimately, the ego is just an illusion. A mind-created fantasy. A mental illness, an insanity that keeps peace trapped in a cage in the soul of each human being.

However, there is a shift in consciousness happening on a greater scale than ever before in human history. As evidenced by the many contemporary teachers throughout the world that are living today. And the spread of that consciousness, the spread of the end of identification with ego, with form, with thought. And the arising of presence and being and divine, pure consciousness, not only in spiritual teachers, but in the many lives that they are affecting throughout the world. Ordinary teachers, students, professionals, factory workers, corporate executives. It's happening everywhere. As the madness of egotistic consciousness brings us to the brink of destruction, the light of consciousness is arising in greater and greater light than ever before. This is the hope of humanity. This is the hope of humanity.

When you begin to study these teachings and learn about the shift in consciousness, the ego will react. I don't want that. That's poppycock. Don't believe in that. We cannot afford this not to happen. We cannot afford to allow the egotistic consciousness to continue, to rein in this world.

Where does it all start? It has to start as a revolution—or an evolution—a shift in consciousness in each individual. That is ultimately the only way that it can happen until we become one family of humanity, rooted in being, emanating with peace and love, knowing that we are all connected at the most fundamental level. Knowing that we are one energy, one life, one timeless eternal life. Until we realize this in the marrow of our bones, in every cell of our bodies, in the deepest corners and reaches of our consciousness, we will never find peace until we know this at that level.

And if we know this at that level, how can we ever hurt another human? Hurting someone else, attacking someone else both physically or psychologically, is like attacking our own selves. It's insanity.

So there is still hope for humanity. But that hope lies in the quiet revolution from ego to presence. Bring being a prisoner of past and future psychologically to being and living now. This moment. All there ever is. Life itself. One eternal life. When this revolution of heart and consciousness begins to reach the leaders of the world, the political leaders, the business leaders, the academic leaders, all of those people who are in positions of influence and power, then we can see a change, a permanent change, from madness to sanity.

Until then, do not put your hopes or your beliefs or your dreams in the promises that are based still on ego. New agreements—will never last, nothing that is unreal will ever last. Only the real is eternal. Only the real lives on. Anything that is not real never lived. It has all been a great delusion, a great dream, a great drama. Shakespeare said, "All the world is a stage." And we are just actors. We are puppets in the world of ego.

But the time for that show, is it over? The final curtain is happening. The final act is playing itself out. In Revelation, it talks about the new heaven and new earth. And the destruction of the world. This will not be physical destruction of the world. All that is needed to transform this world into the kingdom of heaven is the shift in consciousness. When every person throughout the world can wake up every morning and the light and the peace and the love of being and presence, the divine energy shines forth through their eyes and awareness and their words and their deeds.

You may ask, How can I contribute to this peace? How can I become part of this revolution of consciousness? The most important thing to remember is finding yourself, your true self beyond the level of mind and ego. It's not an achievement; it's not something that you do. Otherwise it's still trapped in the world of thinking and doing. Fundamentally, we are already ourselves. We are already that being, that consciousness, that pure divine awareness. It's trapped in the depths of our soul. It's covered up by the mind, by the thinking, by the ego.

So how can we liberate that from ourselves? Jesus said in the Gospel of Thomas, verse 70, that we can only save ourselves by knowing who we are and allowing that to come out. And if we don't, we will surely die. This was taught to us two thousand years ago. Yet all we want to think about is our own salvation—me, me, me. It's time to think about humanity as a whole; since we are all one, we all need to be saved.

So fundamentally you are that consciousness, but the mind and ego has put you to sleep. So we need to wake up. This is all of humanity's wake-up call. So how do we wake up? It's one simple process. We need to recognize that we are not our mind and our ego and our bodies. We need to solve the fundamental human identity crisis. Once we recognize this, and once we can recognize the ego in ourselves, once we can see it clearly by witnessing our lives, by being the witness, not the thinker, but the witness to our own lives, once we shine the light on that egotistic consciousness, it will lose its power because ultimately it's not real. And that is how you deal with the darkness. You cannot fight darkness. But you can eliminate darkness by turning on the light.

Today there are many contemporary spiritual teachers who are bringing that light in the tradition of all the great past spiritual teachers, and they're bringing a light that is so powerful and so divine that the world will definitely change. So when you wake up in the morning, ask yourself this question. Am I part of the problem? Or am I part of the solution? Each one of us has within our own power to be part of that solution, and we don't need to learn how to think differently or to do differently.

We need to learn, as I said in the previous chapter, to be our true selves, to live rooted in the present, in the now, in being. And from that place, we will have right action. We will have right thoughts. When you live from that place, it's impossible to sin. It's impossible to create conflict or misery on other human beings.

And this is not just about stopping wars between nations, the Iraq War, and other conflicts throughout the world. It's also about stopping domestic violence, the battering of women and of children. The sexual abuse of children. All of these things are acts of violence. The criminals who will steal and rob and murder. The arguments of politicians, defending their position as right versus the left is wrong. The egotistic madness of today's political situation here in America and elsewhere.

What do you propose, Congressman? Well, I oppose this. Well, I propose this. Well, I'm opposed. Why? Because I'm on the other side of the aisle. If you're a congressman or senator, ask yourself this question. Are you living from being? Are your thoughts and actions in Congress really for the sake of humanity? Not just for the sake of America; we need to go beyond that concept. America needs to transcend its own collective ego. We can never liberate the world through the propagation of simple democracy. Unless America transcends its own collective ego. There is a better way. Let's stop the madness everywhere. It's not that difficult.

We need to recognize who we are not. And when we recognize who we are not, when we peel away that which is not ourselves, and we disidentify from that grip of ego, what we naturally are will shine without any effort, without any doing, without any thinking.

We've all caught glimpses of this state of mind and this state of consciousness throughout our lives, and many times we don't recognize it. When suddenly we come upon great beauty in the world—at the top of a mountain, by the ocean, a beautiful sunset—and deep inside of us something goes,

"Wow! Amazing!" Our mind stops briefly for a second or two. And being is shining through.

When a great sportsman is playing his sport—hitting many home runs, scoring touchdowns, acing in tennis, shooting a 59 on the golf course—this isn't done through thinking; this is not a product of the ego. This is being shining through. The zone, they call it the zone. In the zone. All of us need to get in the zone, in every aspect of our lives. Not just brief glimpses here and there. We all need to be in the zone. The now. This moment. As the great Zen masters have always taught us: no mind. No mind. The only question is, can we and will we get there? It may seem to the mind to be impossible. When you're in the grips of the mind, the compulsive conditioned thinking, not only as individuals but as humanity as a whole, will make you feel trapped. You could not feel peace. How can you? You're possessed by your own mind. But that's not who you are.

If you want peace in your own life, in your family, in your community; if you want the joy of being, then this is the way. Buddha taught it 2,600 years ago. Jesus taught it two thousand years ago. Mohammed and many of the other great leaders of those spiritual traditions, many of the great Indian sages, Ramana Maharshii, and many others all point to one essential truth, which cannot be expressed in words. The words are just pointers. The words are just signposts. They're the limited expression of the eternal timeless truth that is beyond words and language.

Don't get stuck on the signposts. The signposts are there to help you realize who you are. To know who you are. Not to believe in something so that you can gain reward in the future. This is not ultimately going to liberate humanity.

The time for faith and belief is over. We need to know and realize who we are. One consciousness, one life. God's children, whatever you want to call it. And whatever name you want to use. That's still the level of form, of words. Ultimately, that's not where God exists, or whatever name you want to use—stillness, presence, nothingness, Brahmin, Allah, Jehovah, Universal Prime Energy. Words don't matter.

Deep down inside we all know this. Let's stop fighting about it. Let's stop getting bogged down in theological dogma. It's meaningless. Wasted energy. Wasted consciousness. Even science is pointing us to the same reality, the quantum physics.

Let's stop the debate of evolution and creationism. These are still just battling on a level of thought. It doesn't matter; they're both true. Humanity has evolved; the world has evolved over millions of years. But it has been guided by that one consciousness. The formless, unmanifested ground of being out of which everything exists. The space around the room, the awareness I am. Before I am anything, I am. Let's stop the madness once and for all. We can do it. We're all in this together. There is no "them." There is only "us." There is no "time." There is only "now." There is no "death." There is only "eternal life." There is no separate me, there is only life itself. We are life itself. All of us.

Conclusion

Most people internally have a relationship with themselves. On both sides of that relationship are I and myself. I like myself. I don't like myself. I can't live with myself. I'm proud of myself. And so on and so forth. Talking to ourselves. What humanity needs now is an exorcism of myself from the I. We need to realize that we are not two, we are one. When you look at both sides of the equation, what is real and what is an illusion?

When we realize who we are, the I am, the awareness, to be true, the myself then becomes the illusion. Me, myself, and my story. So what is the tool of this exorcism? Do we need a priest? Do we need holy water? Do we need a cross?

No. How can we perform this exorcism on ourselves? Each human being needs to be exorcised of the egotistic consciousness at the fundamental level. We need to basically take a shower and clean off the ego from our divine essential radiant being. We need to wash off the obscurations, the misperceptions, the dirt, anything that keeps us from radiating our true, pure, divine nature. The shower is basically recognition. The spiritual shower of recognition. We need to recognize that I am. We need to recognize that dimension in our life that is beyond thinking, doing, becoming, acting. The deep inner knowing that is beyond thought. That is the fundamental basis of peace in the world. That is the liberation. This is what the Buddha spoke of; this is what Jesus spoke of. This is who they were. Fully realized, divine nature.

However, that's who we all are. And if your mind ever says that's impossible, then you have forgotten who you are. And once again, the ego has covered up and won the game, won the dream, put you into the dream world again.

This is a spiritual wake-up call for all humanity. Recognize. Be true to yourself. Be honest. Recognize your own reality. Open the door to the depths of your soul. There is nothing to fear. This is simply going back home. Going back to where we came from. Going back to the source. Going back to our original nature.

If you sense any fear in this, recognize it as ego. It is illusion. It is the mind's attempt to survive. It is the ego's attempt to hold on as the dream of illusion fades away and the light of your pure consciousness radiates and grows stronger and stronger.

As the clouds part, as the clouds dissipate, as the fog lifts in the morning, and the sun arises and shines, let that be your internal world. Let that be your liberation. Then we will see a new heaven and earth. We will wake up to the reality of this world. The reality of the earth. The reality of the cosmos and the universe. And for the first time be able to see it in its pure essential reality.

So let go of the little me. Let go of the illusion. You don't need to fight. You just need to recognize. Turn that light on so the boogie man in the dark that's been haunting your soul will wither away into nothing. Amen.

Part II

**Conscious Awakening
Now and Forever**

Introduction

If you look at human history in terms of content as well as the teachings of all the major religious and spiritual traditions, they all pointed to one thing: that there's a fundamental dysfunction in humanity. What we're going to discuss, the conscious awakening, is how mankind in general can identify and transform themselves away from or out of that dysfunction and reach the full human potential originally created by life in humanity.

Let's start with the fundamental dysfunction itself. Humanity is suffering from the spiritual identity crisis. What exactly does that mean? If we look back 2,600 years ago, the Buddha taught us that there was a problem with the self or that there was no self. What exactly does that mean? The meaning is simply this. For some reason, our original ancestors lost their identity. Or better characterized, they misidentified themselves and have been searching for thousands of years, through the various generations, to find themselves throughout the ages. This identity crisis has to do with the original ancestors' dysfunction. And although we may not know exactly how it happened, we do know the results of that.

Humanity suffers from the problem of not knowing who they are at the deepest level or the essence of themselves. When you look at the situation, there are two aspects or two dimensions to live. In Buddhism, it's called form is emptiness and emptiness is form. When I was young, I studied Buddhism and I read that concept. Form is emptiness, and emptiness is form. And I couldn't understand it. But now I understand it clearly. What does it mean?

Just like there are two dimensions to any form, for example, the room that I'm sitting in now. There is the actual form itself—the walls, the chairs, the rug, the table, the television, my body, my thoughts, my emotions—everything is in this particular room. But there's one other element that most of us miss. And that is the space in which the room exists. Without the space in which the room exists, there would be no room. There would be no form, there would be no thoughts, there would be no emotions.

The same is true for our lives. Without a perceiving consciousness or awareness, there would be no form for our lives. It wouldn't exist. We would not see anything, we would not feel anything, we would not think anything. We simply would not exist without the awareness or the space that allows for the forms to manifest.

So what is the identity crisis? The identity crisis is simple. Mankind has never known itself as that awareness. Most of the great sages and mystics, spiritual teachers of the past have all pointed to this fact, but somehow humanity has missed this point very clearly. And wound up finding themselves lost in identification with form, thinking that they could find themselves in the forms. In the material forms, in the physical body, in the thoughts, in the emotions, which are just other types of form in the world of form.

And you see it very clearly. When someone owns a car, they would think of it as "my car." And if somebody hits "my car," we feel a sense of injury to ourselves. Very simply, we have a sense of investment of self in the form of the car. The same can be applied to the house. The same can be applied to the body, the mind, the thoughts, the emotions. These all belong to me. We have a sense of self invested in these things even though they come and go. The thoughts come and go, the emotions come and go, the car comes and goes, the house comes and goes. The physical body is born. It lives its life—nobody knows how long—and then it disappears. That's the law of impermanence. That's the law of nature.

The one thing that doesn't disappear—that has been there prior to the form, and it continues to exist after the form has gone—is the perceiving awareness, the I am-ness, that allows the forms to manifest. So as such, mankind is aware of the thing-ness of life—the things, the forms—and attempts to find himself and his identity in those things simply because he doesn't know or she doesn't know or they don't know themselves as the perceiving consciousness, which is not a form. It's a pure awareness, a presence, as was eloquently brought out in the book *The Power of Now* by Eckhart Tolle, and numerous other spiritual teachers throughout history.

This awareness exists. This is always with us; it never leaves us. It can never leave us. It is the fundamental ground of who we are, which allows the forms of our lives to manifest.

And because of this dysfunction, we feel a need to create a substitute for that loss of identity. Henceforth the ego is born. The ego is nothing more than a mind-made entity. As Tolle puts it, "a mind-made entity, a bundle of thoughts and emotions created by the mind because of its lack of understanding of who we really are at the fundamental essence."

In other words, the ego possesses us, takes us over, creates the story, creates the so-called experience of our lives without being rooted in life itself, in the awareness and understanding and perception through that awareness.

So what is conscious awakening? Conscious awakening is a process. Some people call it enlightenment. Some people call it awakening. Some people call it finding their true selves. Whatever name you put to it, it's basically a transformative process or experience that takes each person out of the ego mind or ego consciousness and into the awakened mind or the awakened consciousness. In other words, we wake up to who we truly are. We find our true identity. We're no longer lost in the world of form, whether it be material form or thought form or emotion or experience. Form. And this process has happened to numerous people throughout humanity, but it's happening more and more on a broader scale than ever before in the history of humanity.

So what we're going to focus on in this book is basically the process, the experience, and the fruits of awakening. In other words, from my own experience as well as the experience of studying numerous other people that have had this happen to them at some point in their lives, or in the midst of the process currently. We're trying to understand exactly the nature and phenomenon of this experience and process. And also try to understand the fruits of that awakening.

In other words, how are our lives different once we have gone through this process of waking up? Are there different levels or different degrees of wakefulness? In other words, is it all or nothing?

I heard a comment recently at a meditation gathering I was at. One person asked the teacher, who is a guru from South Korea, this question: Can you be a little bit enlightened? Or is it like being pregnant—it's either all or nothing? You're either pregnant or you're not pregnant.

And traditionally, it's been viewed as a phenomenon of attainment. Somehow you're on the path; but until you're fully there and have attained something, you're not considered enlightened.

In my view, this is fallacy. I don't think enlightenment is something that you can attain. It's not something that belongs at some time in the future; it's something that we realize about ourselves that we already are. By waking up to who we truly are, we realize that we are fully enlightened.

And it no longer has this characteristic of egotistic attainment or some type of achievement or some type of badge to wear or we get a certificate on the wall that says "Okay now, I'm officially enlightened. Everyone look at me, I'm special."

No, the process is really about discovering what is there and has existed from the beginning of time, and has existed from the beginning of our own birth, discovering our true divine humanity deep in the recesses of our soul and our mind and our spirit. Deep down below the surface level of the forms in our lives.

If we use the analogy of the ocean; the forms of our lives—the thoughts and the emotions and the experiences, the physicality—are like the waves on the ocean. They come and go. Sometimes turbulent, sometimes calm. But our identity belongs in the depths of the ocean where we are unmoved in the stillness of our soul. This is where our true identity lies.

So this book is written primarily to start explaining or beginning to help people understand the process of conscious awakening—the experience of conscious awakening, not as some type of formal commitment to attain something in the future. But it's like peeling away the layers of the onion—peeling back the ego mind, identifying, recognizing, shining the light on it so that it loses its power and its grip over our identity.

We start by identifying what we are not. We are not our body. We are not our experiences. We are not our thoughts. We are not our possessions. By pointing out and recognizing what we are not and understanding when the ego is still in control and shining a light on that, we're able to free ourselves from the grip and the possession.

The ego is not a personal thing. It's not a personal problem. It's not my ego or your ego or their ego; it's the ego. It's one entity. It's one problem, collective human problem. As Tolle puts it very eloquently, it's a collective human problem. And when someone is totally possessed by the ego, there's nobody there. There's no true person there. It's almost as if an invading horde has entered the person's mind and has taken control of it. And that's why Jesus's words on the cross were so profound when he said, "Father, forgive them for they know not what they do." Simply put, the ego was in control. It wasn't those individual human beings; it was the collective ego.

Chapter 1

Trapped in the Mind, Time Dimension

What's the meaning by the mind, time dimension? Through studying *The Power of Now* as well as other spiritual teachings about present moment awareness, you'll find that the core essence of reconnecting ourselves through our true identity is the ability to develop and cultivate present moment awareness.

This comes from the fact or realization that there really isn't any such thing as time per se. You know, when we look at a clock, we think of it as some type of time, that there's some kind of stream of little itty-bitty moments happening one after the other in a continuous stream of time. But in reality, a clock is just a mechanism that ticks and ticks and ticks. Time really exists in one eternal moment, which is the now.

The now is something that we can never get away from. We always experience life in the now. The now never changes. It never moves. And it's one place where the ego cannot survive. Because the ego is not real. It's not life. It's a pseudo form or pseudo entity that traps us in the time-mind dimension.

If you think about it, whenever you're thinking about the past or the future, you're really not there. You're really not aware of life. When you're obsessed with anxiety and worry and concern about what's going to happen tomorrow, what's going to happen a year from now, what's going to happen ten years from now, your mind is lost in a world of illusion and delusion. It's exactly where the ego wants it to be. That's where it can feed on its own existence; that's where it can keep itself alive. That's where it can survive in ourselves. That's where it can maintain a position of dominance and control over the individual.

Or when we think about the past, worried about what we did in the past, reliving the bad experiences, reliving the hurt of our childhood, reliving the pain of accidents and mistreatments and losses that we had in the past, we are trapped in the time-mind dimension.

And, unfortunately, this is how most human beings live, being pulled from one side to the other. The future and past. And future and past. And future and past. With brief glimpses of the present moment. We wake up in the morning, and the sun comes out. We see the sun rise, and our mind stops and we go, "Oh, that's so beautiful." Or we're in an accident, in a car wreck; or we're climbing a mountain, and we're at the place where the danger and the imminence of death is so real that the mind stops and all we can do is focus on the present moment. Or that of a sports player in the zone where they're not doing it through their mind; it's just flowing through them from the present moment awareness.

We have these brief glimpses, and many times we don't even realize. Another time is when we talk to our pets. We never talk to our pets through the ego. We never talk to the pet and put on an air and pump ourselves up and try to show the pet that we're better than them. It's always our pure innocent original mind.

So there are brief glimpses of the now, of the present moment, where the ego cannot live, where it suffocates. But normal human beings, normal human life is being pulled from one extreme to the other, trapped in the time-mind dimension.

So how can we liberate our self? How can we go beyond this? What can we do?

First, we must recognize. Recognition is the key. You can't fight it; it is what it is. But when we recognize it, all of a sudden we create space and we create an awareness that is no longer part of it, that brief moment when we recognize and we step back. When we witness that dimension, that phenomenon in our life is the first step out of prison. That's the key, the key to unlock the prison door.

Chapter 2

Liberation in the Now, Immersion in Presence

It's like we said at the end of chapter 1. The key to escaping the mind-time dimension where the ego thrives is present moment awareness. That is the key. That is the only place where we can step out of that dimension, and into life, the life dimension. The aware, awakened dimension.

If you look at ancient spiritual teachings, for many thousands of years, they all come down to this central point. We need to witness our lives as an aware presence. We need to step back from being immersed in the form reality of our life, which is not reality; ultimately it's illusion because it's impermanent. Nothing remains. Everything is constantly changing. If you take a look at quantum physics, it will tell you that the thing that is sitting here in front of you—the vase, the chair, your physical body—is not solid. It's not solid, it's not permanent. It's always changing. I think, what they do say, that the cells in your body are completely different over a seven-year cycle.

So you are not the same person you were seven years ago. You are a totally new entity, on the form level. You are not the same. You are constantly changing. Form is ultimately impermanent. The teaching of the Buddha, the law of impermanence.

So cultivating presence. Cultivating present moment awareness. This is the key. Witnessing, meditating, which is another form of witnessing. It isn't setting a time aside and saying, "Okay, I'm going to meditate" and experiencing even deep meditation and then coming out of it and then going right back into egotistic mind. That's not the ultimate way to go. It's like getting out of prison and going back into prison—getting out and going back in. You're on a furlough maybe when you meditate. And then, oh, time's up; back to prison. Here we go.

Ultimately, there is no separate time for meditation. Meditation has to be 24/7. Moving and unmoving. It's finding the stillness—every moment. Because there is only one moment. There is no moment to moment. There are no multiple moments to life; there's one eternal moment.

And when you start to experience presence as a reality, you realize that it's deep. It's endless. It's almost like being immersed in water. You stick your toe in and get a little taste of it and then you get further into it and then all of a sudden you want to completely immerse yourself in it, into the depths of the ocean. That's where the liberation is. Go down and stay down.

It's not a path of higher and higher achievement in the egotistic sense. It's actually an immersion into the depths of your true self. The depth dimension of yourself. If you were to prescribe a physical direction to it, it's down. We're going down. We're pulling, being pulled in by the gravity of life: the spiritual gravity is pulling us down.

When Eckhart Tolle talks about his transformative experience, he talks about being sucked into a vortex of energy that's pulling him down and a voice talking about letting go and not being afraid. It wasn't about achieving higher and higher states of enlightenment on the path through some ultimate graduation ceremony. It was about going down, getting down into the depths of our innermost self. The immersion in presence. At first it might be through technique, but ultimately the technique will drop away.

In the Hindu teaching, you have Brahmin, which is God; Shiva, which is awareness; and Shakti, which is energy. Or another way of putting it is, wisdom, spiritual insight, awareness, and energy. Consciousness and energy. So in the immersion in the now, we need to approach it from a three-dimensional point of view. If you take a look at a table, you need three legs for it to be stable.

So insight and wisdom don't always have to be traditional spiritual teachings. It could be from literature, poetry, anything that points to the dimension beyond form.

Consciousness, awareness, meditation, deep meditation, different things that can help you with meditation—there are new meditation techniques available now that are based on audio that help you meditate deeper and quicker and immerse yourself in the deeper state of mediation quickly. Ultimately, you're rooting yourself in the now. You're rooting yourself in the being of who you are.

And then finally, some type of body work or energy work—whether it be yoga, traditional yoga or tai chi or something that will make alive the flow of energy within you, the feeling, the sensitivity to the flow of energy within you. Immersing yourself in the now. Immersing yourself in the present, in being. Rooting yourself.

You know, in Buddhism, in Zen, they talk about rooting yourself or grounding yourself so that your center of awareness is not in your head. It's not trapped in your mind, in the constant possession of thought. It's in the point just below the navel, the groundedness. The spiritual gravity pulling you to the center point. It is ultimately pure awareness, pure consciousness, pure nothingness beyond form.

And indeed, it is nothing. It is no thing. What does it mean, nothing? The meaning of nothing is no thing. How can it be a thing? If it was a thing, it wouldn't be life. If it was a thing, it would be just another form. It's the space from which all things manifest and come from and ultimately return to.

Chapter 3

Tipping the Scales

When we look back on the history of enlightenment, we can see that there are rare occasions when people have become enlightened in a dramatic, totally transformative process. It is very rare; occasionally, it's happened. There are some ancient spiritual teachers, enlightened masters awakened, fully awakened in an instant, in a moment. In a nanosecond. Plunged completely and totally into presence never to return, never to be trapped again, never to struggle with the ego mind.

But on a broader scale today, there are thousands and

thousands of people all over the world who are waking up. And for the most part, it is a more gradual process. From a chronological viewpoint, it seems to have some time involved in it, but it's really not. Because all there ever is exists at the present, for one moment.

In my own experience, I got a taste of it. It was a pretty dramatic taste. I had come to a place in my life where everything that I had attachments to that I felt who I was, that I identified with as myself, was the year 2002. Every aspect was challenged or threatened or lost. My marriage, my health, my career, my financial situation, my home, my mental health, my company. Everything was uprooted in one eight-month period. One damn thing after the other. And this came after years and years of striving for success and reaching for the stars and trying to live the American dream, which I met for many years. I debated writing a book about it, "American Dream, American Nightmare." How the escalation of the culture of more, wanting more, needing more, pursuing more, the endless egotistic spiraling, going out of control, striving for success—never quite getting there, never quite being satisfied, always looking for more, wondering when am I going to make it. Getting to the point where you think you've made it and realizing it's empty. It's a dead end. Why? Because forms never last. Success will never last. It's always changing. Good fortune sometimes and then decline. And then reemergence. It's like being on a giant roller coaster. Up and down and around and around. And right back in the same place. And let's go again. Let's go again.

How many times do we need to go on that roller coaster before we say, "I've had enough, I want to get off. I want to step off." This is how life, which is the ultimate spiritual teacher, brings us to the door of the prison and gives us the key to get off the roller coaster. To get off the merry-go-round. To stand on the sideline as a witness and watch all the various forms in our life take place. But when you're off the roller coaster and you're watching it, it's a totally different viewpoint than when you're on it.

So my experience began at a crisis point in my life when all I could do was just let go, just give up. I had reached the end of the rope, the proverbial end of the rope. To the tenth degree. I had gotten to the point where I could not shut off my mind. I had to go get some drugs from a psychiatrist to try to shut down my mind. I was so obsessed with solving my perceived problems that were just compounded and grew at a greater and greater scale—as I had more and more success, I was more and more stressed. I had more and more fear. I would wake up in the middle of the night in a fetal position, shaking with just unbelievable waves of fear. And I would think about waking up in the morning and knowing I'd have to drag myself out of bed, get in the shower, get ready, and go back to the office for another day of it. Another day of torture. But what could I do? I have a family to support, an image to uphold. Thinking that I'm on the path to happiness. I'm on the path to success. One day we'll get there. I don't know when, but if I just try a little harder, it will ultimately come. False hope and false faith in a perceived future moment that would never ever come.

And then through the spiritual teaching of *The Power of Now*, one day after I had decided to let go, to give up, in total exhaustion and frustration, I was in a bookstore looking for an answer, looking for a new direction. Looking for something, I didn't know what. Walking around the religious and spiritual teachings section.

I had as a youth been involved in a new religious movement and had dedicated myself for many years to it before I got into starting a family and having a career in the financial planning world. So I had an experience with spiritual awakening as a youth and dedication to a belief system and some kind of new world and new age and the dawning of a new age and the changing of humanity. And our group was going to be on the forefront of doing that, of making that happen. Still, future. All about the future. Arriving at some moment in the future. Working endlessly until the age of thirty, I was dedicated to that. And then I finally reached the end; I couldn't do it anymore. All the promises, all the hopes, all the dreams just became shallow and empty, as nothing panned out and nothing really happened the way we all thought it was supposed to happen.

Then losing myself in the world again, back in the world. Starting out a career at a late age, feeling like I had to catch up. Feeling like I had to make up for lost time. Started from scratch. Nothing in the bank, just a lot of desire and determination. I learned a lot during those times as a missionary about the power of intention, the power of determination, the power of perseverance. The ability to transcend the limitations of the body and the mind by just undaunted determination and faith; things would happen. This was the reality of God for me at the time. Faith and commitment to make things happen. I learned many things during that period of time.

But here I was, forty-five years old and spent, emotionally and spiritually, physically exhausted. Yet, still with the responsibility of family, career, a heavy burden to carry every day. I would go take a shower in the morning, and I would feel totally negative. Every cell of my body just filled with negativity and dread. To the point, sometimes I just couldn't get out of bed; but I dragged myself and threw myself in the shower, and I would turn on the cold water and try to shock my body out of this misery.

And it worked occasionally, for a brief moment or for a few minutes, or for an hour or two. And then ultimately the heaviness and the descent of that burden. All the time smiling at work and pretending everything is okay and feeling like an empty shell, feeling like a hollow person, just totally hollow. Nothing on the inside. A facade. And if the slightest little thing went wrong, just ready to explode, ready to detonate. Ready to lash out. And having those feelings happen and then trying desperately to control them. The torture of the mind and the ego.

And then one day in this bookstore, all of a sudden there was the book, *The Power of Now*. I'd heard something on television. This book was famous, that it was good, and so I said, "Let me try; let me see what this is about." And I took it home, and I read it. I couldn't put it down. It was like something was speaking to me in the bottom of my soul. And my mind and heart and spirit just opened completely. And I felt tremendous relief, tremendous peace. Answers to the questions, to the difficulties. Here it was. I didn't figure it out in my mind. But somehow life had sent me a life preserver, a life rope. And I had a very profound experience and I felt a deep sense of peace come over me and I felt this spark of joy in my life again.

But it wasn't a total transformation. It was a taste. It was the first meal in many that would follow. And I found myself a year later in a similar situation, not quite as desperate but related to my career again. The company closing down and a seventeen-year career being uprooted and thrown to the wind, and I found myself struggling again with my identity. Who am I? What's going to happen? The fear and anxiety of the future.

But I'd been studying the book and reading other books by different Indian and Buddhist sages including mystic Christianity. My mind was thirsty for it over and over again.

So anyway, one evening I was particularly struggling with this issue of another career crisis, feeling restless, and anxiety and fear arising in my mind again. And I was sitting in my living room; it was like two in the morning. I couldn't sleep. And I opened the book again, *The Power of Now*, and I turned to a page. I just opened it; I hadn't particularly looked at where I was going to study, look at the table of contents or anything. I just opened it. And I began to read the section on the pain body. And how to make it conscious and how to transmute it from fear into peace.

And I said, "That's interesting. Let me see it. Let me try this." And instead of resisting the fear and struggling with it and fighting with it, I allowed it to be and surrendered to it. I made it present. I made it fully conscious in my soul and my being. I felt it completely. I faced it head-on. And in a few minutes, after feeling it completely, I felt it move from the bottom of my body all the way up through my torso and right out the top of my head, like something had been released. Like an energy had just shot up into space, into wherever. Out of my body. And I felt this fear just go. Completely. And then again, a deeper sense of peace came over me, that was very profound. Very, very beautiful, actually.

And I can actually say from that moment, which was about two years ago at this point, I have not felt fear of anything. Any kind of situation, any kind of thing that happened in my life, I have felt a complete lack of fear, even with things that used to scare me. I used to watch horror movies and science fiction and things that would make me feel scared. And I see those things now with no effect. It's like it just goes right through and nothing sticks. Completely flows through me.

And as I've studied *The Power of Now* and listened to many videos of Eckhart Tolle talk about death and dying and the profound spiritual practice of contemplating the impermanence of life and ultimately your own death, and I can honestly say that when I think of those things, I don't feel fearful anymore. I don't feel any sense of fear about it. And my only explanation and answer to that is when you touch the eternal dimension of yourself and you realize that your life is not a form but it's beyond form, then what's there to fear? There is no death. There is no time, there is no death. There is no them. There's just one eternal now. And it's all of us together. We're all in it together. We're all in the same ship. Floating through eternity.

So let's get back to the topic in this chapter, tipping the scale. So it doesn't necessarily happen in one profound movement. It's like a scale. And as you learn from life and as you experience life and as you practice the teaching, the meditation, the wisdom, the body movement, it deepens. And the scale goes from being heavy on the old mind, the conditioned, unconscious mind, the egotistic mind patterns, and the waves of that hitting you, and that lessens and lessens the weight of that over time as your presence grows and develops. And your scale begins to tip in the favor of presence. It becomes deeper and deeper.

And through the teaching is one thing. That's very important. Points you in the right direction. It gives you the ability to recognize within yourself. It gives you the ability to make conscious what is unconscious. But then through the meditation, and I've particularly been practicing the audio meditation, the accelerated meditation with the audio technology which I find to be tremendous. It's almost like adding gasoline to the fire—tremendous sense of rootedness and presence through that practice every morning, of at least an hour. And then more recently getting into the body movement and yoga and the energy, sensitivity to energy and live energy.

It's gotten to the place where presence is dominant—totally dominant. Where you start feeling no sense of time, just blissfully living in the present moment, watching the forms of life come and go in your job, in your family. Not that you're totally emotionally detached, but you're feeling life fully. You're experiencing the vivid reality of it.

I guess I still struggle some with eating. I love to eat and many times it brings me into unconsciousness so I've ordered a CD about conscious eating to try to help with that issue with me. But it's tipping the scale. It's moving toward the right direction, toward the spiritual gravity.

And then also realizing it never ends. There's no end to it. There's no beginning, and there's no end. There's no graduation ceremony at some moment in the future. Just give that up. I talk to a lot of people. They tell me how hard it is to become enlightened; how you've got to strive, and you know, maybe after forty lifetimes and all your karma has been transcended—consumed or eaten up—and now you're ready. But as Eckhard Tolle said, "You only need time if you think you need time." Until you realize that you don't need any more time. That there is no time. There's only now.

So this has been my experience of tipping the scales. Going from getting a taste of it to allowing it to be and allowing it to grow and flourish and watching through recognition and practice and meditation, it deepens and deepens and deepens. And the sense of peace and joy and the sense of evenness with the things that you do, the quality of those things, of attention and awareness, in my business as a financial advisor, having the ability to really listen to clients and really give them that awareness, is so important. And they feel it.

You know, whether or not you know everything about investments or insurance or planning or retirement, the main thing in this business is serving the client. And understanding and empathizing. And looking for the best solutions for them. With a sincere mind, having no hidden agenda, having no egotistic sense of a means to an end, the client is a stepping stone to my own success. Simply being there to purely help them has added quality and dimension to my livelihood that I haven't had before. I thought I was there, but I wasn't. I was a mixture of altruism and egotistic future success domination.

So for most, the arising, the awakening is a process of tipping the scales. It's not about being in a flash of an instant, like a Vagra sword. I'm sure some people have that experience—but for me it wasn't.

Chapter 4

Freedom from Thought Possession

Let's examine this a little further. There are two dimensions to life. Let's step back a moment; let's take a look at this. So there are two dimensions to life: the form and the essence or formless or consciousness. The awareness. Out of which the forms arise.

Let's categorize this in the human condition. Most people are, once again, trapped in the ego mind, on the surface level of consciousness, identified totally with form. In a sense, it's a form of possession. There's an entity, it's called the ego. It's not my ego. It's not your ego. It's not personal. It's the ego. Possessed by thought. As Descartes said, "I think, therefore I am."

But in reality, he had it totally backward, totally reversed. It should be "I am therefore I have the ability to think if I need to."

If we believe in "I think, therefore I am," then we are possessed by thought. Thought is the dominating factor; thought is controlling our lives. Or upside down. We're moving away from spiritual gravity; we're moving away into the world of illusion and feeling no roots. The Bible talks about the tree of life. Adam and Eve cut off from the tree of life. Exactly what we're talking about here. Cut off from the source of life. Which is now. So in the state of conscious awakening, we are able to reestablish that connection to the tree of life, to the root. Rooted, grounded in the now, in the being, in the presence. Whatever term you want to use. We have basically performed an exorcism of thought on ourselves. Through the arising the presence in our innermost being, it is liberating us from being possessed by thought.

In other words, our consciousness is arising above thought. No longer trapped in the dimension of mind and time. Pure awareness. It's not falling below thought; it's not becoming unconscious through sleep or intoxicants or some type of addiction. Because we're trying to relieve ourselves from the torture of the mind. It's rising above thought. It's consciousness without thought. In Zen, it's called no mind. One of the main Zen teachings is no mind, no problem. No, mind, no problem. Pure awareness.

What a liberating thing to feel. When you have the ability to be above thought, to use thought when it's necessary, when it's practical; when you need to do something, when you need to take care of your life situation. But to realize that you are not your thoughts. Your sense of self is not invested in the thought. My this and my that. This belongs to me and this is my possession and this is my belief system and this is who I am. My thoughts. What a liberation to be able to sit and watch your thoughts as the witness. With the space between the awareness and the thought.

You think of your mind as the open sky, the deep blue sky, or the night sky. And your thoughts are just the clouds moving through the sky. Or the stars twinkling in the night. And you're aware of the space, that dimension of awareness. That is freedom from thought possession. In Hindu, it's called detachment. Nonattachment. We're not attached to our thinking. We're not attached to our emotions. We're not attached to our experiences. They come and go. They float through our life, just as water runs down the river. As the water flows down from the top of the mountain, as the clouds pass through the sky. This is freedom. This is the transcendence of form into the timeless dimension of now. Eternity. Eternal life.

Jesus didn't say to the disciples, "Listen, guys, I'm going to be betrayed by you, they're going to nail me to a cross, I'm going to die, and your liberation is by believing in me." He never said that. Jesus pointed to the real solution. The kingdom of heaven is within us. And you must save yourself through that realization. This is what Jesus taught. It's in the Gospels, if you look beyond the traditional Gospels. It's in the Gnostic Gospels.

Jesus was in the desert for forty days. And ultimately Satan came to him and said, "I will give you all of this." He showed him all the kingdoms of the world, all the possessions. "I will give you all of this if you bow down and worship me."

And what did he say? "Get thee behind me, Satan."

In today's contemporary spiritual terminology, let's look at that. The kingdoms of the world represent the world of form, the world of thought, the world of emotion, the world of possession. And in that act of renouncing Satan and renouncing those things and refusing to bow down, he basically rose above thought, into pure consciousness.

The kingdom of heaven is within us. We are the kingdom of heaven. We are the awareness, the witnessing presence, that's rooted in life.

Most people have a relationship with themselves. There's I and myself. This was the beginning of Eckhart Tolle's liberation. His life had become so heavy with the burden of self that he finally realized he couldn't go on any longer living with himself. And then he said, "Wait a minute. Am I I, or am I self? I can't be both. Am I one or am I two? I have to be one or the other." And that became the beginning of that transformation.

So do we really need to have a relationship with our self? Does a dog have a relationship with himself? Does a monkey sit in a tree and contemplate, 'If I do this, how is that going to be? How is it going to affect my self-esteem? What if I do that?'" No. They are simply themselves. One entity. One consciousness. One awareness. There isn't an I and myself.

This is freedom from thought possession. Give up the relationship with yourself. It's not essential. There's no need for self-esteem. If we are already complete and perfect, why do we need a relationship with our self? We already are complete. Lacking nothing. So give up the relationship with yourself. That's true freedom.

Chapter 5

Freedom from Time

We've already alluded to this in other parts of the book. But when we enter the awakened mind, the awakened consciousness, and we're liberated from the mind of ego, the time-mind dimension, we develop a sense of freedom from time. Where does that sense come from?

Well, in reality, there is no time. Time is an illusion. Psychologically, there is no time. The future and the past are simply illusions. They're a mental concept. We never experience the future; and we never experience the past, except as mental thought forms. What does that mean? There is no time. It doesn't exist. There is only now. And the now is eternal, timeless.

Again, what a sense of liberation to know that we can rest in the now through that pure awakened consciousness and be freed from the pull of time. If you go to a busy street in a major metropolitan city in the United States and ask people, "What are you doing? Where are you?" Most of them will tell you, "Well, I just finished a meeting over here and on my way to the airport because I'm going to the next meeting over there." Their life is an endless stream of being pulled through time, psychological time, mind projections. Past and future. They're not present; they're not here. There's nobody there. They're unconscious. Trapped in the ego time-mind dimension. Cut off from the tree of life. Living in the world of good and evil; the tree of the knowledge of good and evil. Mentally judging and labeling everything. A conceptual reality that has nothing to do with ultimate reality of life itself.

So through the awakened consciousness, there will be a growing sense of freedom from time and liberation from time. Time will be used in the chronological sense in terms of planning, learning from the past and planning the future. But not trying to find our sense of self and identity in those dimensions, which ultimately don't exist, except for thought forms.

It's okay to plan the future, to try to map out a direction for your life. Your life situation. But again, once we know ourselves, our true identity, we're not looking for ourselves in the future, which is just an illusion. It is just a thought form. Then we'll never be disappointed because we know it's not there.

One of the most profound stories in *The Power of Now* is the first story about the beggars who were sitting on top of the box that was full of gold worth ten million dollars. They didn't realize what they were sitting on. They were putting their hand out all the time looking for something, looking for a solution outside themselves all the time sitting on that box of gold. The gold being metaphorically the true peace and love and joy of being.

So through the awakened consciousness once again, we develop the sense of freedom from time; of actually going through and living your life in a timeless dimension, in eternity. When we know ourselves at that level, we know we are eternal and we know time does not really exist. Time has stopped.

Some evidence of that is when you're talking to some of the successful sports figures and they talk about being in the zone, say in a football game or a baseball game. What do they all say? "Well, it seems like the game slowed down. Everything was in slow motion. I was able to see and perceive things in a different dimension."

That's what happened. Did time really slow down? No. They're beginning to realize there is no time. Ultimately, there is no time; it's an illusion. There is only now. We experience every moment of our life as now.

Chapter 6

Freedom to Choose

What do we mean by freedom to choose? Through the awakened consciousness, when our complete life is made conscious, then all the unconsciousness—the past pain, the conditioned thinking, the repetitive conditioned thinking that many times we're not even aware of, the habitual patterns of action that arise out of conditioned thinking—when all of that is made conscious, then therefore liberated, we are put in a position of freedom to choose. Freedom to choose to do the right thing, or what Buddhists call correct thought, correct action.

Because how can anyone commit evil from the position of an awakened conscious mind? When the choice is obvious, there is no choice in reality. It is an impossibility for a fully awakened, conscious person to do wrong. Because when you're awakened fully, you feel the connectedness to everything in the universe. Every form, not just the people, but the things. The animals, the trees, the flowers, the plants. All the forms of life. You understand the essence, and you understand that that essence exists in everything and we're all part of it.

Even scientists have proven now what Buddhists have said for over two thousand years ago—that there is no separate anything. Everything is all interconnected in one flow of energy. And the totality is making reality as it is.

That's why it's futile to resist the suchness of life and the is-ness of life. It's futile to live trapped in the time-mind dimension of egotistic consciousness. It's ultimately just wasting your life. Because you have no life. You are life. You might as well join the team. You might as well jump off the merry-go-round. Get off the roller coaster. Give yourself the freedom to choose. The freedom to choose the path that makes the most sense that springs forth from the joy of being and from the root of life. How can that be otherwise? How could that create anything other than oneness with the whole? Ultimately, it's not even your choice. You will choose life.

Yes, but the world is full of evil, isn't it? The world is full of humans inflicting pain and suffering on other humans and on animals and on nature. Isn't that real?

Ultimately, no. It's human unconsciousness. It's ego manifestation. The ego desperately trying to hold on to it's self sense of identity of who it is, masquerading as good and bad. Good and evil. It's nothing personal.

So through the awakened consciousness, we develop true freedom to choose.

Chapter 7

Freedom to Do or Not to Do

If we are already complete and whole, as we are, because we realize ourselves, then what do we need to do? Do we need to do anything? The answer is ultimately no. We just flow aligned with life in the now, without any particular need to accomplish or to do or to act in any way—immersed in the joy of being alive and the happiness and peace that transcends the polarities of good and evil, right and wrong, pleasure and pain. All those things that we feel are so real and so a part of us when we've been living in the ego mind.

It also means the freedom to do if we consciously choose to do. But that doing will have a quality like never before. Fully awakened, fully conscious, full attention. Not doing in the egotistic sense of an ends to a means, making the present time into a means to an end. Looking for something in the future. We will do out of compassion to enhance the lives of others because the lives of others are our life. The same one life. We're not really doing anything for others, we're just doing them for ourselves. The extended self. The one life, the polar opposite of the ego.

So the question is really a matter of possession. Who's in possession of your identity? The ego or the one life? Jesus said, "You cannot serve God and serve mammon." You're either trapped in the one dimension or you're master of both dimensions of form and consciousness. Or at least you're moving in that direction.

And this point is very important for all those people out there who are so consumed with doing and accomplishing something all the time. Achieving something. Ultimately if you're not doing from being. In other words, what comes first, being or doing? Most of us have been trained from the ego perspective that in order to become somebody, we must do something first. We have to achieve something to be somebody.

Once again, just like Descartes with "I think, therefore I am." We've got it all backward. That's not the way it works. Being is primary. I am. First and foremost, before I am anything. And before I am doing anything. I simply am. Myself. And from that place and from that rootedness in being, if something bubbles up and springs forth in terms of action or doing, it will be imbued with a sense of quality like never before. And the ultimate result will be taking care of itself simply by doing and by being. That doing won't have some ulterior motive, or a stepping stone mentality.

And this sense is all enhanced through different types of

meditative practices like the vipassana meditation, the awareness of the breath and the body, and the walking meditation where we're taking steps not for some future goal or expectation but simply to be totally aware of each step in the process. One after the other. Raise one foot and set it down. Raise the other foot and set it down. Over and over again.

When we look at humanity, we see people who are possessed by doing. Got to be doing something. Well, what are you doing? People call up on the phone, they say, "What are you doing?" "Well, I'm doing this. What are you doing?" It's all about doing. It's not about who they are. It's not relating to each other as one pure consciousness to another, which is ultimately an illusion anyway—it's all one consciousness anyway. Well, what are you doing? Well then, what are you doing?

We gain our sense of identity and selfhood by what we're doing. Today I'm going to work. I'm working in the financial planning business. I am a financial planner, that's my sense of identity. And that's true, but that's not your ultimate identity; that's your form identity. Or that's your profession. Instead of saying I am a financial planner, I could say, my profession is financial planning. That's how I make my livelihood. But that's not who I am.

I could also say I am a father. I have three kids. But that's not who I am. That's my form identity. That's my life situation. What we are is just so much more vast and deep than that.

I am, therefore I have the ability to think if I need to. Being comes first. I am. Therefore I do. If I choose to do. And I don't do if I choose not to do. And it doesn't really matter that much.

As conscious awakening happens, the natural ability for compassion will grow in you without even trying. Because you feel the connectedness to everything. And if you feel the connectedness, you're going to feel the compassion to help anyone in need, to take care of them just like you're taking care of your own body. Ultimately, we're all part of one large body. One interconnected entity sharing this whole universe.

So let's not get trapped in doing and thinking that we must do. And feeling uncomfortable if we're not doing anything. I know people who just can't sit still. They're so restless because they're so uncomfortable with being. They're so identified and habitually trained and conditioned to do that they could never relax. They could never just hang out one day and read a good book or sit around and watch the sunset and watch the grass grow and watch things happen in the home and just be aware of it.

So it's like John Lennon and the Beatles when he finally gave it all up and said, "I'm just sitting here watching the wheels go round and round. I love to watch them roll, no longer riding on the merry-go-round." Just had to let it go. There's a lot of wisdom in that. Playing those mind games.

So the freedom to do or not to do. Whatever you choose, make sure it's coming from an alignment with life. And how do we align with life? We align with life by surrendering to the moment. By surrendering completely to the suchness of this moment. Because this moment is reality. This moment is what life is. Life itself. And more importantly, that's where the connection is.

We're all like big screen TVs with no antennas. We can't get the signal because we either have no antenna or we have a broken antenna. The signal is there; it's beaming down from the satellite all the time. The sun is shining all the time, but the clouds are obscuring it and blocking it. Our antenna is broken. We need to get replugged in. If you pull the plug out, all the juice goes out of the TV. We've lost the animation. We've lost the ability. We're just a blank screen.

That's what life is like in the ego mind. Emptiness. Loneliness. It feels like a big hole right in the center of your heart. And we've become obsessed with trying to fill it up, not knowing that on the other side, there's another hole where it's just going right out the back door. So we think if we work harder and collect more and add more and do more things and be more and become more and achieve more, and you know, save the world and recruit everyone to our particular belief system or way of viewing things, following the new, you know, new age guru, the messiah, whatever you want to call it, then somehow that hole is going to get filled up. Never happens. Can never happen. It's an impossibility. It's not going to happen.

We need to wake up to the reality that we don't need to do anything to be ourselves. Why would you need to do anything? You already are yourself at the essential level. You are totally complete. Already one with life. Divine nature.

I get a kick how people make excuses for unconsciousness by saying "Well, that's human nature." That's human nature. That's human weakness. Human nature is divine. Original human nature is divine. There is no gap between humanity and divinity; it's one. The gap only exists if you create it in your mind. If you create the gap. If you conceptualize and put God in the concept and put him up from you so far away that you can never reach there.

Same is true with Jesus or Buddha or anybody else. If you worship them as idols, you're creating your own road block, in terms of your own realization. When Moses went up to the mountain and came back down from receiving the Ten Commandments, the chosen people that God had prepared for hundreds of years were worshipping a golden calf. Have we them our past saints and sages and religious pioneers and the heads of the great religions and turned them into golden calves? Or more correctly, has the ego done that? Has the ego created that obscuration, that road block?

There isn't anything you can do that matters that much. Ultimately, what you do matters but only in a relative sense, as it relates to your life situation.

Chapter 8

Rewiring the Brain, Locking in the Gains

In previous chapters I've alluded to a technology called audio-enhanced meditation. And there are a lot of different products on the market, but I guess there are differences in qualities and effectiveness. But the one that I've been using has worked extremely well.

This technology is based on scientific research that was started back in the '70s when the first wave of Eastern gurus came to America and taught transcendental meditation and other forms of meditation to young people and students throughout the country. The research was done by basically placing electrodes on the brains of various yogis and meditators and analyzing the brainwave patterns of various states of meditation at the deepest levels.

Basically what they found was, as a meditator meditated deeper and deeper, their brain waves changed dramatically—the patterns changed, they slowed down into various rhythms or waves. Ultimately going from the beta wave pattern, which is what our normal waking consciousness is in our everyday life, to alpha and then theta and then finally to delta, which is similar to or the same brain pattern for dreamless sleep that we all experience every evening when we go to sleep; when we've gone beyond the dreaming, the rapid eye movement sleep, into the dreamless sleep.

So what does this actually do for your brain? Well, your brain is an ever-changing organism—constantly changing, constantly creating and disconnecting different neurotransmitters and neurons and different connections. And it's dependent upon your experience, what you experience in life—depending upon the input.

Through this study they found a certain type of audio stimulation with a difference between the left and the right ear. If it was done appropriately, it would basically force the brain to adjust and to harmonize between the left lobe and the right lobe of the brain.

Most of us experience life as either left-brain dominated or right-brain dominated. Studies have shown that. And there's not a lot of communication between the two sides of the brain. But apparently this technology, and I've read some of the literature and the books associated with it, creates more communication between those two sides of the brain. So what does that actually mean?

It means that instead of looking at things in a divided fashion—and dividing and judging good and bad, right and wrong, left and right, and perceiving the world through a divided kind of brain function as the brain works together and harmonizes more—you tend to look at things from a holistic point of view, as an integrated, holistic viewpoint.

And as this develops and this happens, and your neurons are being rewired, you develop the ability to deal with more input and more stresses without the brain getting overloaded and shut down. There is more emotional resilience. You don't react negatively when difficulties that come with the circumstances in your life create too much stress. The brain has the ability to deal with it.

It is amazing that more people don't know about this. Apparently this one particular technology that I'm using has been used and tried by several hundreds and thousands of people all over the world. And I'm quite amazed that it's still not as well-known or as widely known. I guess there's a lot of skepticism in some areas of the psychological community about this, but I have to tell you from my experience that it definitely has a tremendous impact.

If the brain is already being rewired constantly as our life experiences change, what is so hard to believe that we can have some impact on that through different technologies? We live in the era of technology. And some of those technologies are wondrous and have changed our lives dramatically.

I mean, up until one hundred years ago, roughly speaking, humanity lived in a very, very different way. Life expectancies were much shorter. Medical technology hardly existed. Advancements in power, communication, travel, medicine, and the various technologies (computer, digital) have come about over primarily the last one hundred years and have changed the world dramatically. We no longer live in a vast world; we live in a global community. The ability to speak to someone on the other side of the world—by phone or through the Internet or by e-mail and to be able to travel from one side of the world to another within a matter of twelve hours or so—has shrunk the world down tremendously.

So in the area of spirituality and meditation, why wouldn't we also take a look at advancements in technology that could help humanity accelerate the pace and deepen the experience of meditation? And the multiple benefits that could be reaped by that advancement. What are we afraid of? Science has proven—the various studies over the last several decades—that meditation is beneficial for the health in many faceted ways. Yet most people find it extremely difficult to meditate on a consistent, regular basis because without any kind of added support or technology, it's a long and can be a very frustrating process. To be able to get through the chatter of the brain, the mind-made me. The little egotistic entity that is sitting there waiting to catch you and to keep you from exploring the depths can be very difficult.

Now there are different techniques of meditation that can be helpful. But I believe very clearly that the audio-aided meditation is a way to help people meditate at a very deep level without really much effort at all. All it requires is to sit and listen. So some commitment of time and some commitment of listening and that's it.

As a matter of fact, according to the book I read regarding this, even if the person falls asleep, the brain is still being rewired because it's still receiving the stimulus through the ear. And the difference between someone who stays awake and conscious during that meditation session and someone who falls asleep is very little.

So what does that mean? Well, that could mean that we can actually meditate while we're also asleep and have similar benefits and similar effects. How much easier can that get? But from my own experience, the depth of stillness and peace that I have experienced through this has been tremendous. It's almost like adding fuel to the fire.

But at times, there have been things that have come out during the meditation. Different images or visions or emotions, unconscious feelings that have come out and have been released that I'm experiencing has been extremely beneficial. And apparently this is what happens as the brain gets stimulated at deeper and deeper levels and your brain wave patterns change and do the various stages and then remain at the delta stage. Your unconscious becomes conscious.

So this is truly a scientific method of conscious awakening that we're looking at here, not just some kind of airy-fairy spirituality that people have difficulty relating to. But actual scientific evidence and scientific technology that can help humanity awaken. And I'm still just at the beginning of this. I'm about eight weeks into it; and I have to tell you, it has added fuel to the fire when it comes to my experience of presence and being awakened, living a fully conscious life.

So my proposition is this. I wouldn't say that the audio technology was the beginning of my awakening—certainly it had its roots in a spiritual teaching. The beginning of which was the actual, the ultimate spiritual teacher which is life itself and the life circumstances that seem to force us at some moment to change, to transform—as life itself helps us to break down the shell of ego and to crack and open and transform ourselves.

But this isn't a moment in time that just happens once and it's over. Or a state of attainment. Now we've got it. Like I said before, I've got my graduate certificate in enlightenment now. Everybody, I'm special. This is not the meaning. It's opening a world of endless depth. There is no bottom to the pit. But there's nothing to be fearful of the pit. The pit is where we came from. The deeper you go, the more benevolent you feel.

So if we can have this deepening, through the variety of methods—and I hate to use the words *method* or *technique*, but through the combination of life experience, spiritual teaching, meditation, energy body movement, yoga, all these various methods so to say—and through the audio technology, we're able to rewire our brains to lock in the gain. This also is very beneficial.

So as we go down, as we become more and more attuned to the spiritual gravity that's pulling us down to the center, into the vortex, back to the source of life, the tree of life, we are able to apply scientific technology to lock in those gains. What a marvelous thing. A way of preserving and protecting the fruits of this awakening.

The particular technology that I've been using is something called Holosync which is available through Centerpointe Research out of Beaverton, Oregon. I've also read the book of its founder Bill Harris. I have also listened to some of his retreat workshop audio CDs. This technology is definitely making a substantial contribution to this consciousness evolution that humanity is going through.

And after having been through my experience as described earlier in the book, I am excited to realize that I'm still at the beginning level of the program, of Holosync. I'm still at the prolog. There's actually twelve other levels that you can go at your own pace. You can go as far as you like in the program, and stop at any time. It is up to you! I am just totally excited to go through this and to see what unfolds.

How are we living? It seems to me that we've only just begun. Einstein said something like even the most advanced brains in the world still have only used about 20 percent of its capability. So what are we waiting for? Why are we allowing our limited beliefs to keep us down, to keep us trapped in the mind-time dimension of egotistic consciousness? It seems to me that we can use these technologies to really make advancement.

It's almost like the planet itself is crying out for this change; that we're living in a moment in history that is a pivotal crossroads for humanity. If you look at the history of humanity, it's a flat line until the twentieth century. And all of a sudden, it's a rapid ascent into development.

The same thing is taking place on an internal level. The outside is just a reflection of the inside. The madness and the egotistic consciousness are getting more and more severe on a daily basis. We see evidence of that throughout the world. But at the same time, on the internal side, there is an arising of consciousness, on a scale never before experienced by humanity. As evidenced in the book *Translucent Revolution* by Arjuna Ardagh, the awakening is happening to all types of people. Professionals, workers, blue collar, men, women. There is no discrimination. There is no egotistic sense of worthiness so to speak. It's happening, and it's happening to thousands and hundreds of thousands of people throughout the world. Maybe it is time for a new heaven and new earth.

Chapter 9

The Real Self

What do we mean by the real self? The true self, the divine self.

As I was continuing to record this last chapter on the real self, my daughter approached me and reminded me that she needed a ride to school, to Driver's Ed that morning. So I stopped the tape, got dressed, and took her and her friend Elena to school. One thing to notice about this was an interesting experience. It is extremely cold. It's December 14, 2005, and it's extremely cold. And when I went out and got in the car and sat in the car with my daughter, it's one of those mornings where the car just doesn't warm up that quickly. And I could feel my body contracting, and I could feel some place in my mind, the desire, or this inclination to complain. And my body contracting and shrinking. Becoming small.

What's that have to do with the real self? Well, let's think about it. The world of ego and the egotistic consciousness is a cold world. It's ultracold. Because there's no life in it. It's a phantom. It's totally empty. It has no central substance. It's basically a fictitious identity that we've created because we don't know our true identity. It's something that is always searching for completion, to add more to it. Or to complain. It can only live and survive if it traps us in the time-mind dimension, away from the now. The now is not its friend. The now is where it becomes suffocated and ceases to exist.

So it's very helpful to understand our real self by understanding what we are not and identify what we are not. Now some people who might be reading this who are still pretty much identified with the mind dimension, the ego mind, might say, "What does that mean? The real self. I don't know what that means. What's that all about? Explain that a little bit more. Give me some detail. I want to understand this. I want to grasp it. I want to hold it. I want to smother it."

But for those who have tasted or begun the journey of conscious awakening, the real self is no more than just a waking up to what we already are, what we truly have been all along, but have been covered over and obscured by the mental possession of the egotistic mind.

So let's do a little exercise. Maybe if we can identify what we are not or we can identify where we cannot find our self, ultimately what will be left is our self.

I am not my material possessions. I am not my physical body. Ultimately, the physical body dies. It's a temporary home for my true self.

I am not my thoughts. My thoughts come and go. If I

believe and acted on every thought that popped into my mind, I would be categorized as a schizophrenic maniac. All of you know that you've had thoughts in your life that when you caught yourself, said, "Wait a minute. Why am I thinking like that? Where did that come from? I can't do that. I can't be that." It's almost shocking, sometimes, the things that pop into your mind. Is that who you are? I don't think so. These are just thought forms that pop into consciousness and go away, drift away. But they carry with it an emotional energy, an emotional charge, which brings us to the next point.

I am not my emotions. My emotions are triggered by those thoughts. So I am not my emotions.

I am not my experiences. A lot of people are addicted to experience. This experience and that experience. They're not interested in finding themselves beyond their experience; they just are addicted to having multiple experiences. Let's try anything. Jimi Hendrix asked, "Are you experienced? Are you time tested? Have you traveled? Are you a person of the world? A man of the world? Seasoned and salted by the endless stream of thinking and the endless experience and emotion and roller coaster that you're on?"

The next question is, are you experienced in the present? Are you experienced in the now, in living in the eternal one moment of the now? Beyond the time, beyond the form?

So we are not our experiences. We are not anything. And I emphasize the word *thing*. Just as things come and go, our identity cannot be found in the form level of existence. It's an expression of our true selves, but it's not who we are. I am not anything. What does that mean? Well, if I'm not anything, that means I am nothing. And to the egotistic mind, that is uncomfortable. What do you mean, I am nothing? I am this, I am that. I did this, I did that. I look like this, I look like that. How can you say that? That's crazy. This is all poppycock.

But indeed, we are nothing. Indeed we are no thing. Because beyond the veil of form, is the world of no things.

Buddhism called it the nothingness. The void, the emptiness. The illuminated light of emptiness.

So if I'm no thing, then what am I? I am consciousness. I am awareness. I am being. I am presence. I am the now. I am. Life is a journey to find our identity at the deepest level. And when you start that journey and you go through that journey and experience that journey, which is not a journey of time, it's an immersion in the depths of eternity.

That doesn't make you special. As a matter of fact, if you think you're special, then you missed it. You're heading back toward the ego mind. The ego would like to tell you that it's impossible to live like this. You'll never attain it. You'll never achieve it. You'll never be there. It wants you to buy into that limiting belief, the toxic concept, that it is something that's going to happen in the future, something I have to strive for and work toward to become worthy of something.

But that's not what it is. And one tradition of Tibetan Buddhism is the concept of *dzogchen* that simply means resting and settling in our natural self, of who we are.

You may have had an experience with this already in your life. I'm sure you have. Almost everyone does, except they don't recognize what it is. It comes and goes.

Where do you find it? It's captured in the brief moments of pure alert consciousness without thought. It's captured when you're sitting with your pet and you're talking to your pet without any pretension or egotistic masquerading.

It's in the moments when you feel the tears, the joy, the expression that you can feel from the bottom of your heart and soul when you are exposing yourself to the world or to your closest friend or to a stranger in an act of kindness that is beyond any calculated ulterior motivation. Pure, kind compassion that wells from the bottom of your soul, that spills out into your life in a variety of ways.

Life, as I've described it here, is so beautiful. Indescribably beautiful. It is 180 degrees different than the ego madness that most of humanity lives in. Looking to the future to add more to me, to this little entity, to feed the ego. And once again, remember it's not my ego, it's *the* ego. It's not who you are, it's an imposter inhabiting your body and your mind.

And the funny thing is, when the truth of this hits you in the marrow of your bone, it's almost as if you've known this all along. It's almost like you've been living with amnesia—thousands and hundreds of thousands of years of human amnesia. Don't know who we are. So instead of looking where we should, in the depths of our own mind and our own soul, for our true identity, we've been seeking it in the forms of the world. We've been playing the game, we've been living the drama and not ever realizing that we are the audience. We are not the actors on the stage. We are the audience.

This is the real self. This is who we are. This is who you are. The one life. And when you have that realization, you lose the sense of separateness from other people. You feel a deep connectedness to everything and everyone because that's who we are. We are that present, aware consciousness that we share. It's an amazing realization.

If you look at the vast universe and cosmos and the multiple forms of life on the planet, even within our own solar system, the amazing phenomena, and you realize that whatever power, force, energy, consciousness created this whole universe, I am a part of that, and that created me. The same awesome, unimaginable depth of awareness, creativity, insight and wisdom, intelligence, and energy not only created me, but that's who I am. That's who we are. What an amazing realization.

So that's something that we cannot find outside of ourselves; that's something that we cannot find at some point in the universe. The answer lies within us. We have to go back to the source. Joni Mitchell said back to the garden, "We have to get back to the garden."

Jesus said that the answer lies within. It is in all of us. How could it be otherwise? It cannot be otherwise. The self. The I am. Before labels, concepts, and forms obscure that, that is who we are.

So how do we enter that dimension? And this is again directly from *The Power of Now*. And it's so simple; it's almost like, how can humanity have been lost for so long, when the answer is plain as day? But think about the beggar sitting on the box full of gold. The answer is really simple.

We have to surrender to this moment. Completely. Because this moment is where life exists. Where that connection is. This very moment, which is not just a flickering time-bound moment; it is the eternal moment, timeless and eternal, that has unlimited depth. Surrender to it now. You'll never find it in the future. Because when the future comes, it will be the now. The future and the past do not exist. Only as mental forms. Surrender to the now. And see what happens.

This is the ultimate key to unlock the prison. Many years ago, Ram Dass wrote the classic *Be Here Now*. The pointers have been out there for centuries, all pointing to the same thing. Yet we have never listened. Only a few individuals ever listened to life's calling. Life has been calling us back. Back to our home, for centuries. It's time now to listen.

Conclusion

Conscious awakening is happening to all of us. How, you might ask? Wherever you're at, whatever you're doing, you are surrounded by a spiritual teacher. It's called life itself, which is the ultimate spiritual teacher. And by whatever means necessary, that we can't even understand because we're too busy judging our lives and other people's lives, other events and experiences from the egotistic perspective with—I wouldn't call it rose-colored glasses—the distorted, maniacal glasses of ego. But even in the midst of that, life is gently and sometimes severely educating us and pushing us back to the present moment, where we have the ability to liberate ourselves.

It could be through a spiritual teaching; it could be through a meditation practice, prayer, whatever means necessary. Prayer is more of a subjective plea to God for something. We need to listen. How do we listen? We need to meditate, not just in a sitting, formal way, but as a witness to our entire life as we go through our day. We need to listen to the inner voice that is calling us. But are we listening?

And it could come to us from deep inside; it could come to us as we meet a beggar on the street. The realization, or even something they may say to us, may be exactly what we need at that moment to bring us back.

That's what life is. The ultimate intelligence. But it goes so much further beyond intelligence than we can imagine. It's also the ultimate emotion. True emotion of peace, joy, and love. That is endless in its depth and its breadth. And it's not bound by the polarities of pleasure and pain, right and wrong. The dual dimension that this world appears to be. It is nondual. It is eternal. It is one.

It could be through religion, although religion is ultimately not necessary. The purpose of religion is to ultimately destroy itself; to make it unnecessary to be religious. Most religious people get stuck on the signposts, thinking that the truth is contained in the words or in the teacher alone. That the teacher—Buddha, Jesus, Mohammed, whoever—has a monopoly on God. That it is in sole possession of God. Therefore, we could never have that. Therefore, we need to be religious, stuck in religion.

Let's not get stuck at all. Let's not get trapped in a belief system that ultimately will be controlled by the ego. You want to be liberated—liberate yourself. Find yourself, your real self. It's right under your nose. It's nowhere else. It's deep in your mind. Let it come out. Let it be. The Beatles said, "Let it be." "And in my hour of darkness, she's standing right in front of me, speaking words of wisdom, let it be."

Let life be. Align yourself with life. Surrender to the now. Do not resist. Whatever form your life takes, whatever happens, allow it to be. Surrender. Find that peace in surrendering. And then see what happens.

So once again, conscious awakening is happening to all of us. Are you ready to get off the roller coaster? Are you ready to give up success in the egotistic sense? The pursuit of the phantom that you can never grasp. So stop trying. Stop chasing your tail. If we could step back and look at ourselves, we would see that we're just a little dog or a little ego chasing its tail around and around and around. Never getting anywhere. Thinking that we're getting someplace.

We are already there. No need to look any farther. No need to look outside of ourselves. Doesn't exist outside of the self.

Part III

**Incarnations of Life:
Search for our True Identity**

Introduction

When you look at the history of humanity throughout time, and if you were to plot that pattern on a graph, you would see that for most of the recorded history, human beings lived in a very simple way. They were born, they grew up, they developed a skill or trade, they worked that skill or trade, and then they died. And that was the pattern of human life for centuries.

Yes, there were kings and leaders and things in history that were the exception to the rule, but for most human beings, they lived a very simple life. They very rarely traveled farther than forty or fifty or sixty miles from their home. Their knowledge of the world, the knowledge of the universe, the knowledge of anything beyond their small sphere of life was very limited.

And so if we take a look at the teachings of Hinduism and of reincarnation, the basic philosophy has always been that the human being lives a life span—they grow to a certain degree, and if they haven't attained enlightenment in their history of life at any point, they die. They go through the *bardos* of death, only to reemerge, possibly as a new human being, in the process of reincarnation.

And Hinduism says it takes many multiple years, even thousands of years and thousands of reincarnations in order for that person, or that spirit, to eventually achieve or become fully awakened and enlightened. We look at that basic principle or phenomenon, and we apply it to the modern age. It may seem that something has changed dramatically. Once again, if we put that human history on the graph, we would see a very, very flat line stretching on and on and on. And then all of a sudden, the twentieth century hits; and for some unknown reason, life shifted and changed dramatically.

There are major world wars. There's major travel. The world has shrunk dramatically to the point where it is very common for all of humanity to travel far distances. And to experience things and cultures that were never ever possible, or ever lived, by previous generations.

This has been fueled by a number of things. Primarily, transportation, technology, and today, the information age which has the effect of shrinking the world to a global village.

But what has this done to the pattern of incarnation from a Hindu perspective? Today's phenomena I think is largely influenced by that situation. During one physical life span, a human being actually living multiple incarnations is becoming more and more common. This book is about that phenomenon as it relates to my own life.

During my life, the short forty-nine years that I have been alive in this physical form, there has been a tremendous change throughout the different incarnations. And when I reflect back on it and I look at it, I can see almost totally different people appearing at different times in that life. So what we're going to discuss in this book is each one of those incarnations in those phases. Not necessarily in the mundane detail of how I lived during that time, but essentially what my character was like during those different phases. Ultimately leading to an awakening and an identification with the true identity that we all are, that we all share.

Chapter 1

Altered States

First, let's begin with childhood. I lived a very normal childhood in a small Midwestern community where I grew up with my parents and my two older brothers. And I don't think there was anything exceptionally special or unusual about that childhood. I played sports, I went to school, I was interested in music and things at the time. I went through puberty, started becoming interested in girls, went through all the upheavals of being a teenager. And ultimately grew up in the late '60s and early '70s which was a very interesting time in the American history, with the Vietnam War, the peace movement, and the drug culture that developed during that time.

That wasn't really on the cutting edge or the beginning of that period. I pretty much reached the age of fifteen, sixteen, seventeen in the early '70s, having missed the initial stages of Haight-Ashbury and Woodstock and things like that. I was still young I guess when Woodstock happened. I was thirteen years old. And the idealism and the political side of that particular time had kind of waned by the time I reached fifteen, sixteen, and seventeen years old. The specter of the Vietnam War still hung over our heads, and the threat of the draft was still very much alive. But I wouldn't characterize that period in my life as one of protest or political activism; it was really more on the experiential side when it came to using and participating in drugs. Experimenting with marijuana, hashish, mescaline, LSD, and different psychedelics, which ultimately created a situation where I experienced what I would call altered states of consciousness.

This is very well documented in the life of Ram Dass, who was a Harvard professor. Together with Timothy Leary, he pretty much wrote the book on LSD use back in the late '60s.

So I had a similar experience as Ram Dass, although I didn't experiment with LSD to the magnitude and the longevity that he did. I did have experiences with it that would range anywhere from euphoric, blissful, uncontrollable laughter, hour upon hour. I remember sitting in a Pizza Hut booth one time when I had taken a tab of blotter acid with my friend and sitting there eating a salad and literally laughing. It left me laughing uncontrollably for several hours, as I ate bite by bite of this particular salad.

There were also other altered states that I experienced in that period of time that were not as euphoric and blissful. I visited what I would call a dark side of the human mind. One particular evening, I had gotten hold of some very strong potent LSD that was called window pane. Very, very strong.

You didn't really need to take a whole hit; you could cut it into quarter hits and still go on a psychedelic experience that would last up to twenty-four hours.

I did this with a friend and I'm not going to give his name or really talk about him, except for the fact that we were doing this together and we spent one evening in his home and he got it in his mind that he was going to goof on me. In other words, play mind games with me, tricks, and so forth and so on.

I spent the evening with my friend in his basement, and he would say things to me like, "I'm going to pin you to the wall and brick you in like Edgar Allen Poe's story of 'A Telltale Heart,'" or I forgot which one it was. Anyway, this guy just basically goofed on me and put so much fear in me that I wound up shriveled up and crunched up in a fetal position in a corner, shaking uncontrollably for about three or four hours, until the morning came and I was able to collect myself and get up and go home.

When I went back home and saw my parents, they knew something was wrong; and I knew something was wrong. And I didn't really say anything, and they didn't really ask questions. I got the feeling that they just didn't want to know. I went to my room, and I stayed there all day, trying to recover from this ordeal.

What I found in this altered state, was that the level of consciousness you had going in determined what kind of experience you ultimately had. If everything was good and I was feeling well, and I entered, and I took some type of psychedelic, generally the experience was very, very good. I mean, there were weird things, you know, walls breathing and windows and curtains fluttering and a kind of a heightened sense of aliveness in the world, in the grass and the trees and the birds; kind of a spacey, euphoric, almost surrealistic or being in an impressionistic painting almost. That's what life looked like.

But when you went into that state from a place of problem, where you had things on your mind or issues with other people, normally that would degenerate into a bad experience or what we characterized back then as a "bad trip."

So I went through this for a period of years. I also smoked marijuana, hashish, which were milder forms of that type of altered state. So I know very clearly that there were different levels of consciousness that people could perceive beyond what we'd call a normal everyday consciousness of human life at that time.

So I want to call—besides my childhood being the first incarnation—this incarnation as a kind of the hippie-altered state.

So that's basically the first incarnation. At the age of seventeen, I had gone off to Europe one summer and experienced life on my own, bumming around Europe with my friend and hopefully by myself meeting people and experiencing things. By the time I became a senior, I decided to do that again between the summer of my senior graduation and the plan to go off to college in the fall. And I set out on a journey across the United States and wound up in California. I don't want to go into the details, which I kind of went into in my previous book, but I had what in Christian terms would be called a rebirth experience and in Buddhist or Hindu terms, a Samadhi experience, which was a radical change in consciousness. Not induced by drugs but induced by a spiritual teaching that I encountered through Reverend Moon and the Unification Church.

This Samadhi experience basically lasted for a couple of months, during which I felt total sublimeness, bliss, aliveness, and joy in every cell of my body. And a total oneness with the universe and the cosmos. At that time I didn't know what it was, I didn't know why it happened, except that it did happen. And I decided to join the movement and dedicate my life as a missionary to the bringing of this message and transformation of humanity based on this experience of oneness with the universe.

Before this experience, I had really no conscious belief or disbelief in God. I just didn't know. I would characterize myself as an agnostic. I was raised a Christian but as I got older, found it very difficult to simply believe in the simple Bible stories I'd heard at my parents' church. I had deeper questions about life that just weren't answered in a traditional Christian church setting. And although some of these questions were answered through the teachings of the Unification Church, or back then it was called the Family or One World Family, there were still a lot of unanswered questions.

However, the actual experience and reality of how I felt and what I perceived was undoubtedly real to me in my experience. And it wasn't because I dropped a tab of acid or I smoked a joint. It was natural; it came simply through the pure teaching and experience of the various workshops that I attended when I first joined.

So this I would say would be the beginning of the second incarnation. What I would call the missionary incarnation. And I dramatically changed. I cut my hair. I changed my clothes. I lived as a monk, a celibate life. Lived with very, very minimal food, just basic food, worked many hours a day dedicated to the mission from the age of seventeen up to the age of thirty. Involved with witnessing, fund-raising, business activities. At one point I had become a security guard for Reverend Moon himself. So there were kinds of mini-incarnations in different roles I played in the church. But basically this was my missionary and almost like messianic, evangelical incarnation—my life from the age of seventeen to thirty.

Then I reached a point in that whole phase where I had lost that essence and the church made no more sense to me whatsoever. At least the organization. The teachings were still profound, and I tried to live by the teachings, practice it in my life. But just like any belief system, unless they're bringing you to the reality of the experience, the fresh aliveness of a spiritual life, they just become dogma. Empty, hollow rituals and rules that you follow out of conditioning. And ultimately, I lost that experience. Then I became more and more disillusioned with the organization as a whole, with its leadership and its descent into a collective ego situation, which I felt rather imprisoned by.

No one was keeping me there by force; no one had forced me to join or had trapped me there whatsoever. But more and more, I felt a prisoner of this life. And decided at the age of thirty to separate my professional and business career from my religious beliefs. I kept the Unificationism as a tenet and a way of life, principle teaching. But I was no longer immersed in the movement and working in the organization. I got a job on Wall Street with an insurance company, so basically I started out in the life insurance business at the age of thirty, having come from a totally unrelated background.

I don't know why I went that direction, except for during the time I was a security guard, I would study business and the financial markets as a kind of a hobby. I had somehow developed an interest in that. And eventually when I did decide to look for a separation from the organization in terms of my practical livelihood, it just seemed natural to move to that particular field of the financial service industry.

So I started out as a life insurance agent, did get my securities license shortly thereafter, and went head over heels, full blown into financial planning.

My original job was in the Woolworth building in lower Manhattan, and eventually we moved over to Wall Street so I had an office on Wall Street. And I struggled to do all the practice, to get clients, and to deal with their overall life insurance needs as well as their retirement, college planning, and basic investing needs, at the age of thirty.

And that career has progressed for the last nineteen years, and I have gone through many changes in that particular career. But it also changed my life dramatically. I would call this incarnation of my life the plunge into materialism. It wasn't basically a pure plunge, it wasn't a reaction or a negative reaction against God or against religion; but I simply tried to bring the principles and ideals of my previous faith into the daily life as a financial advisor.

Now just imagine this. You're coming out of a world where it was almost like a monastery, or like a Buddhist monk type of situation, where I had no money, where I lived and worked basically for food and a roof over my head, dedicated to a higher purpose and higher goal in life, not worrying about the future so much, not worrying about saving money. There was no money to save. I mean, at some point, if I wanted to go get a cup of coffee, I had to go beg the accountant, the bookkeeper at the local center that I lived at, for fifty cents so I could go down the street and buy a cup of coffee. That's how strict it was. People had no personal money. Eventually, after we were engaged and married, we were given stipends from the church; but we really lived a very cloistered and very sheltered life, just like you would in a monastery.

All of a sudden, I'm on Wall Street, working in the financial world, the world that is driven by greed and more, the desire for more. The massive desire for ego gratification. And achieving success in a worldly sense. This is the world I plunged myself into. I was going to be different though. I was going to bring the morality, spirituality of that previous incarnation into the financial service arena. And I tried my best for years to do that. But looking back on it, I would say that I was only moderately successful at that.

Now I have been cut loose from the umbilical cord of the protection of the organization so to speak, having to fend for myself, having to make a living, having bills to pay, rent to pay, food to put on the table, a livelihood to make, having absolutely established no credit at all, having no credit, even at the age of thirty. I remember how difficult it was to get my first credit card, And it was a Macy's card. I had to practically beg, borrow, and steal in order to get a Macy's credit card.

Eventually though, as I made more money and I got more credit cards, my credit began to develop and be established. When I bought my first car, I had to get a cosigner at the age of thirty-two. My wife's brother cosigned for the car. But ultimately I was able to integrate back into the regular economics of society over the next few years.

This incarnation, what I've called the plunge to materialism or the financial advisor incarnation, basically has been a very interesting ride. The world of financial services. They are basically producers and nonproducers. If you are a producer, you can make a good living; you can make a killing. And you can go from basically nothing to quite a substantial lifestyle if you really put your mind to it.

I literally started out at the age of thirty with $10,000 in the bank. Now you may say, "Wait a minute, you said you had no money, how did you get $10,000 in the bank?" My wife had been hit by a car at one point, and we received a law suit settlement which gave us a few dollars to start this business. So with that money and a lot of guts and a lot of determination and a lot of drive to succeed, I was going to show myself, I was going to show the church, I was going to show everybody that given the freedom to control my own destiny, I would become successful.

And I pretty much did that. It wasn't easy. There were times when I was, you know, borrowing from Peter to pay Paul in order to stay afloat—in order to run the business, pay the expenses at the business, pay the expenses at home, pay the taxes. It's what I would call a major juggling act to keep this kind of lifestyle alive, really starting from scratch. But in the financial service world, like I said, there are producers and non-producers.

The nonproducers, on the other hand, get washed out very quickly. There was one in particular who was basically a living encyclopedia of insurance investments, financial planning, taxes, legalities, and so forth and so on. However, he never made a dime in the business. Many times I would come in early in the morning and I would find him all disheveled, on the floor in the office, having not shaved or showered, suit and tie all dishelved. because he was desperately trying to break through and to make a living with the knowledge that he had.

But all the knowledge that he had really couldn't do anything for him because he had no people skills. He was insecure and unable to connect with the clients at the human level and therefore unable to sell. And if you can't sell in the financial service business, you're going to starve and you're going to get washed out eventually.

And this financial service business has evolved dramatically since 1987 when I first got involved in it. I mean I became involved in it pretty much two months before Black Monday and the major crash in 1987 in October. Not a real good time to get started in the business. But it's normally a tough business to get started with in general anyway. It was made even that much more difficult because of that severe situation and imbalance that happened in the markets back then. And having said that, the dirty little secret of the financial services industry is the apparent conflict of interest between the salespeople.

Anyway going back to my previous statement, the dirty little secret of the financial services industry is, it's driven by the salespeople. They're the ones out there, selling the stocks, the bonds, the mutual funds, the annuities, the limited partnerships, their life insurance, the mortgages, you name it. The products are out there—the banking services, the lending, the investment banking. And they're basically paid by commission or fee. In other words, they get to eat what they kill. If they can't make a sale, they don't get paid. And if they don't get paid, they starve.

Now put that in the context of the client's side and the regulators' side. It's almost demanding that the salespeople who are driving this industry always look out for the client's best interest and put that first—over their own interest. What a recipe for disaster. What a position it puts the financial representative in. It's almost like let's set up a situation for them where temptation is around them constantly. And let's see what kind of moral character they're made of. And if they slip up in the slightest, if they slip up even one bit, if for one instant they decide they're going to cross the line or they're going to compromise that integrity, the regulators are there to pounce on them and ruin them.

That's one little secret. The other is how difficult it is to run your family and to make a livelihood when your cash flow can be totally irregular—one month you make a lot, one month you starve. Not only the financial difficulty but the emotional roller coaster it puts most people on, especially the tremendous pressure you get as you're struggling to get started in the business.

Now I realize there's not a lot of sympathy out there in the public for the hotshot brokers who make millions out of Wall Street. But that's not the entire financial services industry. There are a tremendous amount of highly ethical, good, solid people trying to make a living, trying to serve their clients, trying to do a good job in the environment that is totally stacked against them. Totally stacked against them. In a world driven by ego and greed and the culture of more. Which quite frankly is driven by our consumer society, which is driven by advertising and media, which ultimately is all an illusion. That somehow you can become fulfilled and have deep and lasting peace and happiness in your life through the constant drumbeat of purchasing more and more of consumer goods and upgrading your lifestyle, getting a bigger house, getting a fancier car, sending your kids to the hottest schools, keeping up with the Joneses, competing with everyone in this endless rat race, which ultimately is a dead end. And how the media perpetuates this illusion somehow in the magazines, in the TV shows, of how the celebrities and the business barons have all made it and they're better than all of us and we need to all strive to be like that or the supermodels are all these kind of influences that we have in our society.

But anyway, getting back to the financial services industry, again, what a loaded gun this is. Clients expect and deserve to be treated fairly and honestly. And they should have the expectation that the advisor is working in their best interest. And most of the good advisors are doing that, the successful ones, because they have built a foundation of success financially where they're not under a tremendous amount of pressure to make the next sale to do that. But that's the exception to the rule. For every successful advisor, there are five or ten underneath them who are having limited success or struggling completely. And there's really no support for those people. It's a jungle; it's survival of the fittest. It's dog eat dog. And in an environment like that, how can you expect to really provide the best possible service to the client?

Well, what is the alternative? The alternatives aren't any better. Let's just do away with financial advisors, and let's basically let everyone do it themselves. Let's let everyone pick their own stocks—everyone buy no load this and no load that, completely do-it-yourself financial management. Talk about a recipe for economic disaster in this country. Yet, that's what the media would have you believe. You don't need a financial advisor—just buy my magazine. Just read my column. The constant drumbeat by the media against products and against advisors, poisoning the minds of the public against them, creating an environment of distrust and suspicion. For what? All so they can sell more newspapers and magazines? Or make a name for themselves in the financial media? So that their TV ratings and their newspaper columns can make money for themselves?

It's a mad world out there. It's a mad industry. It's unbelievable. It's hard to make a living in this country. It's even harder to build a nest egg and retire comfortably and live in dignity in your retirement years, enjoying the fruits of your work. There is a tremendous amount of financial information all over the place. Newspapers, magazines, TV shows, radio shows. Advisors, brokers, financial planners, insurance agents. You name it. Information is flowing all around us, constantly. And what it does is basically create confusion, indecision, and ultimately wrong decisions; peoples' heads are spinning.

What's grossly missing from this equation is financial wisdom. Knowledge that's rooted in experience and working with people and their problems and inserting life planning into the mix of financial planning. And the only way that's going to happen is if you have competent, knowledgeable, and experienced financial advisors who are able to guide their clients through the maze and the bombardment of information that is out there and help them deal with their situations on a practical level as it relates to their money.

And those financial advisors should be compensated handsomely for that. They are the business sages of personal finance. They shouldn't be attacked as greedy, egocentric, arrogant, despicable people that many in the media try to portray them as. The real good ones are almost saints in this world, helping people solve their problems, helping families put kids through college, helping Mom and Dad retire comfortably and live secure with protected income in their retirement. And the great ones not only do that, they also are psychiatrists and psychologists to their clients; helping them to achieve peace of mind and tranquility as it relates to their money and their life. What a noble profession. They are the financial doctors of the world.

So my incarnation in the financial services industry has been very interesting. One of struggle, learning, growing, development. I've seen clearly the inconsistencies and the difficulties, not only for the advisor but also for the various companies—investment companies, insurance companies, banking companies, you name it—as they struggle to succeed and survive and provide the services to the consumer.

This is my third incarnation. It's had a tremendous amount of challenge for me as well on the personal and spiritual level of my life. Which ultimately became so difficult a few years ago that my whole world basically was challenged one particular year. All the structures in my life, I felt like I was losing. My marriage was a problem; my career with a particular company I'd been with for fifteen years became an issue; my relationship with the manager that was above me in that organization became an issue. The business itself had dried up; this was at the height of the bear market. My business was down 40 percent; cash flow was drying up. I had the back taxes and mortgage payment piling up on me. I decided that I needed to possibly sell my house, put it on the market. Found out that I had some health issues that I won't go into details about. One particularly could turn into a life-threatening disease. All of these things came crashing down on me in this incarnation, in that particular year of 2002.

And I got to the point where I basically would sleep very little at night because my mind was racing, trying to find a solution. Trying to break through. It got to the point where I literally could not turn off my mind. It just went from one compulsive thought to the next. Obsessed with getting myself out of this mess. Ultimately, this became almost a psychosis of mental anxiety about the future. That anxiety seemed so great that I literally would wake up in the morning in a sweat, in a fetal position, shaking and consumed with fear, to the depths of my soul. Yet I had to get up, I had to drive into work, I had to put a smile on my face, and I had to deal with my clients, who where either upset about the collapse of the stock market or were sitting on their hands, paralyzed by fear themselves, not doing anything. Which meant to me, that I wasn't going to get paid. *How was I going to pay the mortgage? How was I going to pay for food? How was I going to pay for college?* My children were rapidly approaching the age of college at this point. College tuitions were somewhere between $25,000 to $40,000 a year per child.

Literally, the structures of my world had collapsed on me and were pressing on me to the point where I just didn't know what to do. I wouldn't say I was suicidal, but I probably walked up to the edge of that and took a peek over the cliff.

And then an amazing thing happened to me. I basically shrugged. I said, "You know what? I've been hanging on to this tail of the tiger here, and I just can't hang on any longer. I simply can't handle it anymore." And I decided to let go.

This wasn't really a major change in my business or my profession or anything else. It was more of an internal giving up. I gave up. I couldn't take it anymore. I couldn't live this way anymore. I've had enough. I was exhausted. And I didn't know what's going to happen, but I just couldn't deal with it anymore.

And somehow life turned at that point, in a short period of time, into my friend. As opposed to me struggling with life, trying to beat it, trying to control it, trying to dominate it, trying to make it; I basically surrendered to it. And said, "You know what? You win."

Shortly thereafter, I was in a bookstore, looking in different areas but primarily looking in the area of spirituality—religion and spirituality. Pretty much trying to get back to my roots, longing for the day back when I was seventeen years old when I had that first Samadhi experience of feeling one with the universe, feeling the blissful joy of abundant life in every cell of my body and the depths of my soul. And I wondered, *Where the heck did that go? Where did it all go?*

I knew at that point that it wasn't about making it, or it wasn't about getting caught up on the financial side, preserving my home, getting a bigger home, getting a nicer car. It was no longer about the culture of more and more things. The more forms. The more complexity piling up and piling up on me. I just didn't know what I was looking for.

Then all of a sudden in this bookstore, a book appeared in front of me at the end of an aisle called *The Power of Now*. It's written by a contemporary spiritual teacher named Eckhart Tolle. And I remember seeing that book on the Oprah Winfrey show. I didn't really watch the show much, but I remember seeing something about it on the show. So I said, "You know what? Let me buy this book." And I took it home, and I began to read it. And I read it and I read it and I read it. And it was almost like I was reading my own life story. Page after page, I felt some type of emotional or spiritual release happening inside of me. I felt my awakening stirring in my soul. Questions that I had particularly about obsession with the future and anxiety about the future, being trapped in psychological time; being addicted to the next moment, the next thing—the culture of more. On and on and on. The teaching of the importance of the present moment. Life itself. And being able to live and focus on that. To be present in the moment.

It began to free me from that prison that I had created for myself. And although I still am involved in the financial services industry and I have a thriving practice, that began the latest incarnation in my life—what I'll call the incarnation of spiritual awakening.

Then over the last three years, as I've studied and read, I've probably read that book at least twelve times—it's by my bedside; I open it frequently—it has been a spiritual nourishment for me that has just made a tremendous difference. Life altering. Consciousness-shifting difference.

Besides that book though, I have also now read in the last three years, probably forty other books on spirituality, Tibetan Buddhism, Hinduism, Zen, books by other contemporary spiritual teachers. I've become an active meditator, and I am trying to bring a meditative awareness into my daily life.

About a year after this happened, the company I'd been with for many, many years basically decided to get out of the business and gave pink slips to the over eight-hundred advisors nationwide and said, "Go find yourself a new firm to work with. We're no longer going to be in this business. We're going to focus on our other business, which is property and casualty insurance. We no longer want to be in investment and financial services."

Now, six months earlier, I was inducted into the Ambassador Hall of Fame with that company; and the party was a black tie affair at the Trump mansion in Palm Beach at Mar-A-Lago. So adoration from the company, awards, fifteen years of service, certain amount of business under management, so forth and so on; six months later, "Okay, get the hell out of here. We don't need you anymore. We're going in a different direction."

Which was about two years ago. And again, I felt challenged. I felt uprooted. I felt like my legs were being cut out from under me. Although I had gotten a little bit of a foothold on the spiritual side, I felt some peace or some relief and some development there; once again life had dealt me a blow that I wasn't really ready for.

And I remember literally, again, feeling this energy, this fear, this high-frequency energy in me that was filled with anxiety. And I was sitting in my living room around two in the morning wondering what to do. And I again opened the book *The Power of Now*; and the page I turned to was something called "dissolving the pain body." It explained to me when these types of challenges happen in our life, there are two potential outcomes. They can either make us more contracted, struggle more, and plunge us into further unconsciousness, or they can be an opening to further awakening.

And through the guidance of that book, I was able to work through those issues and that anxiety—make it conscious. Feel it fully. Experience the pain and the fear and move through it. And I literally felt something from the bottom of my feet all the way to the top of my head literally move out of me. An energy, almost a release. Almost like a release of being possessed by something. Lift out of me. Almost like the weight of the world had been lifted off my shoulders. In an actual feeling of energy flowing out through the top of my head. Negative energy. And this tremendous sense of peace, deep peace, just came over me. That has stayed with me ever since that day, two years ago.

And there's probably never been a day since that happened where I have ever felt an ounce of fear. I had struggled for years with depression. I was diagnosed with a mild form of bipolar disorder, which is hyper-mania and then depression after you burn out on the upside; you become depressed and struggle.

Since that day, no depression. No anxiety about the future. No fear. And it's manifested itself in many ways. I mean, I used to watch horror movies, and certain things would scare me. Today I watch those things, and nothing scares me. It's almost like even to the point of the fear of death. Given the thought of death and contemplating death, I don't feel any anxiety or fear about that. Now that may change when it actually becomes imminent. But I feel much more prepared for death than I ever have in my life in the past. And if you look at all of the ancient spiritual teachings about death and the contemplation of death, you'll see that that is the ultimate spiritual practice—the contemplation of the impermanence of life. It's a very fundamental tenet of Buddhism.

So this awakening that happened to me initially back in the fall of 2002 and then the re-struggle a year later has really changed my life. Has really changed my life.

So this is the final incarnation. The incarnation of spiritual awakening.

To further enhance and deepen this understanding of what's happened, I would like to talk about what I'll call in this chapter "The Three Men in My Life." Or another way of putting it, "Three-Dimensional Spirituality."

As I said previously, the most recent awakening that has happened to me in the last several years fundamentally happened because of the spiritual teacher Eckhart Tolle and *The*

Power of Now. It has taught me how to disidentify myself from the form level of my life, the body, the mind, the thoughts to no longer search for myself. The sense of self in the external side of the world, the world of form. But to really seek myself in the depths of my soul in the inner dimension or the awareness that makes the forms possible. In other words, the "I am" side of the equation. Before I am anything, I am. The being side of the life, the fundamental side of life. The essential nature that you can feel through your body and in your soul before you do anything. And before you think anything. And identifying and knowing myself as that.

What a liberation. What peace. To be able to live in freedom from the ego. In freedom from the compulsive, habitual conditioned mind that is running the lives of all of humanity. The collective human ego. I have to say I don't believe I'm totally free of it at this point, but certainly it has lost its control and its power over my life. It doesn't dominate my life anymore. And simply by recognizing it when it happens, the conditioned thinking, the ego, and the games that it plays with other people and situations, simply the act of recognizing it and witnessing is the liberation.

So the first man in my life, this first contemporary spiritual teacher among many—but I would say central to me—is Eckhart Tolle and *The Power of Now*. I studied the book and several other books that he's written—*Stillness Speaks* and *A New Earth*. I also listen to his videos; I also run a silent meditation group centered around those teachings.

The second man in my life is quite different, although essentially a teacher of the same fundamental teaching. And if you really look at it, all religions and all spiritual teachings are basically one. On the surface level, there may be a lot of differences in perspective, in verbiage, in language, which is ultimately not the truth itself. But if you look beyond the surface, you'll find that there is only one truth. But the second man I speak of is a contemporary spiritual teacher from Korea named Khan Ba Da. And I had the pleasure of meeting him over the last several months and experiencing his particular perspective and teaching and practice. And the tremendous power that it has had in the lives of my spouse and some of my friends who met with him.

He also is practicing yoga and meditation. A particular form of yoga and meditation that I will characterize as essential is energy yoga. Which is more of a combination, and it's hard for me to characterize because I'm not an expert in it. But it is a combination of tai chi and yoga. And it's centered on feeling the life energy within us. It's almost like vipassana in the Indian yoga tradition. The meditations through the energy of the body, through the breath, and through feeling the vital energy that's in all of us. And *The Power of Now* teaches the same thing: that the body is a doorway into the spiritual dimension. But he has a practice, and we participated in some sessions with him and a local teacher who's a friends of my wife. And there were several amazing experiences as it relates to those sessions that we had with him.

He also is gifted in the area of spiritual healing and acupuncture. And I saw him give healing and acupuncture treatments (not traditional acupuncture but the simple, specialized, spiritual—I would call spiritual acupuncture) on my spouse, my assistant, and others. And the results were nothing short of amazing. Almost transformative. Energy blockages and mental difficulties and deep-trapped pain, trapped in the unconscious mind, were released through these practices and this energy, the healing energy that he has, that I would say was nothing short of liberating for my wife.

Without going into details, my wife has suffered the burdens of her childhood growing up in the poor country of Korea, losing her father when she was little, having difficulties with her siblings, feeling neglected and hurt, that were built up and had been trapped in the unconscious for many, many years.

These and other issues that are not uncommon with all of humanity because we're all trapped in the egotistic consciousness or egotistic thought-mind level of life. And he basically gave her two treatments on two separate days, and she literally became a new person. Not in the sense of her form or even her personality so to speak, but her sense of joy, her sense of peace, her sense of connectedness, almost like what I experienced through *The Power of Now* in my own particular liberation.

The same can be said for my assistant who suffered for years from migraine headaches, not really knowing why she got them, but suffering with them, taking medication. One treatment of not more than thirty to forty-five minutes and this was all released. And this deep sense of peace and joy, a transformative power, had also helped her in a dramatic way.

So this is also part of my practice, which is the Happy Tao yoga or energy yoga.

The third person in my life is someone I've never met. His name is Bill Harris. And Bill Harris has developed a technology, scientific technology, through the use of audio, that is helpful with meditation. Extremely helpful with meditation. And as a matter of fact, it has the power, on a scientific basis, to help people meditate and develop that meditation much more quickly and rapidly versus traditional methods that are unaided by audio technology.

And I've been going through that program over the last four weeks with what I would call tremendous results in terms of the depth of the meditation and the rootedness in being that I feel because of that. Now like I said, this particular audio technology which is promoted through Centerpointe Research in Oregon, again, I think adds a tremendous dimension in the overall spirituality that I'm experiencing. And this is all rooted in science—it's not just spiritual teaching and concept or even teaching the wisdom of the depth of consciousness. It's also rooted in science.

So I'll call this three-dimensional spirituality. Spiritual teaching, energy yoga, and audio-aided meditation has created for me and helped me develop a rich depth in my life. I hesitate to even say the term *my life*—there is no such thing. There is life. So these things in their own way, in their own faith and form, and by the way, none of these men in my life really know each other. That may change in the future, but they don't really know each other. But each one in his own way has contributed individually as well as collectively to bring me to a place of tremendous peace and joy and freedom.

And I can see it already, the fruits of it in my profession, in the meditation group that we have been developing and with other activities related to them that are developing—almost without any effort. And when I wake up in the morning at five and sit down for my morning meditation, I look forward to that every day. To wake up out of the sleepy dream state, or unconsciousness, into the fully-awakened state of presence and to be able to take that with me into my day. So I start the day with the Holosync audio meditation session for one hour. I usually put on a videotape, the teachings of *The Power of Now* and I'll do some fifteen to twenty minutes of energy yoga and I start my day that way. And I can see it, the quality of life, the quality of relationships that develop, that come from being alive. Not from the egotistic drive of doing and accumulating and possessing life, looking for the future moment, finding a sense of self somewhere beyond the now. The difference is amazing. It's purely amazing.

I am so grateful to Bill Harris, Khan Ba Da, and especially to Eckhart Tolle for their work, for their teaching, for their technology, for their spiritual power. The power of liberation that I know is not really theirs. They are just vehicles. They are just open doors into that dimension. Ultimately, life itself is our ultimate spiritual teacher. The inner guru. In Buddhism and Hinduism, it's called the inner guru. There's the external guru, the spiritual teacher, and there's the inner guru that is within all of us. Because when they teach us, and we have these experiences, it's almost like in the depths of our soul. We say to ourselves, "Somehow I knew that already. It's living in me. It's been a part of me."

And Jesus said, "Before Abraham was, I am." I can really understand that now. The "I am" of my life. The awareness of the forms of my life. The energy, the thoughts, the physical manifestations of not only my body, my surroundings, but the entire universe and cosmos.

Ultimately, that is the purpose of life: to awaken out of the dream into the fully-awakened state of knowing who you are and who we are, who we all are, at that essential level. The fact that there is no "them." There is only "us." One life. One eternal life living in one eternal moment. Sharing and caring and being, together.

These are is the incarnations of life. For whatever reason, the world has changed dramatically. We're living in a time when during one physical lifespan, each human being has the potential to live numerous incarnations and to grow and to be awakened to a new consciousness that really not only can transform the individual but can transform the world.

I hope each one of you can find that, or better yet, can know that and realize that in the depths of your soul.

Conclusion

As we all look back on our past, which has been but a memory trace happening in the now, let us recognize that which was real, the awareness, the I-am-ness that is woven through the thread of those past memories. That which is real is eternal. And that which is not real never lived. Let us sift through those memories and allow the real, the eternal real life, who we are, to shine. And let the illusory egotistic manifestations dissolve away into nothing. Let us allow that to be our practice in the future as well. As the sword of awareness, consciousness, let it pierce through the illusion of the mind and egotistic consciousness and reveal the true reality that is here and now and always will be. Let us walk into the Buddha fields, beyond illusion, into the true reality.

What is the recipe for that? It's very simple. Recognize, allow, and surrender to life. Let life take us by the hand and guide us through to that ultimate reality. Be still and know that I am. Here and now.

Printed in the United States
140048LV00003B/7/A